SLEEP
AND YOU

By the Same Author

Boivin, D.B., and A. Shechter. "Light and Melatonin Treatment for Shift Work." In *Encyclopedia of Sleep*, ed. Clete A. Kushida. Amsterdam: Elsevier Press (forthcoming).

Boivin, D.B., and A. Shechter. "Light Therapy." In *Encyclopedia of the Neurological Sciences*, 2nd edition, eds. M.J. Aminof and R.B. Daroff. Amsterdam: Elsevier Press (forthcoming).

Boivin, D.B. "Jet lag." In Encyclopedia of the Neurosciences, ed. Kate Miklaszewska-Gorczyca. Amsterdam: Elsevier Press (forthcoming).

Boivin, D.B., and P. Boudreau."Les troubles du sommeil et des rythmes circadiens." In *Les troubles du sommeil*, ed. M. Billard and Y. Dauvilliers. Paris: Masson, 2011.

Boivin, D.B. "Disturbances of Hormonal Circadian Rhythms in Shift Workers." In *Neuroendocrine Correlates of Sleep/Wakefulness*, eds. D. P. Cardinali and S. R. Pandi- Perumal. New York: Springer, 2006.

Boivin, D.B., G.M. Tremblay, and P. Boudreau. *Les horaires rotatifs chez les policiers : étude des approches préventives complémentaires de réduction de la fatigue*. Montreal: Institut de recherche Robert-Sauvé en santé et en sécurité du travail (IRSST), 2010.

Boivin, D.B., and F.O. James.*Prévention par la photothérapie des troubles d'adaptation au travail de nuit*. Montreal: Institut de recherche Robert-Sauvé en santé et en sécurité du travail (IRSST), 2002.

Boivin, D.B. "Comment réduire les effets négatifs du travail de nuit sur la santé et la performance ?" Gestion (HEC Montreal) 35, no. 3:47-52, 2010.

Diane B. Boivin M.D., Ph.D.
Foreword by Ève Van Cauter
Translated by Barbara Sandilands

SLEEP
AND YOU
Sleep Better, Live Better

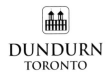

DUNDURN
TORONTO

Editor: Michael Melgaard
Design: Courtney Horner
Printer: Transcontinental

Library and Archives Canada Cataloguing in Publication

Boivin, Diane B., author
Sleep and you : sleep better, live better / Diane B. Boivin
; foreword by Ève Van Cauter.

Issued in print and electronic formats.
ISBN 978-1-4597-2352-8

1. Sleep--Popular works. I. Title.

RA786.B65 2015   612.8'21   C2014-904990-0
                                                        C2014-904991-9

1   2   3   4   5   18   17   16   15   14

 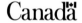

We acknowledge the support of the **Canada Council for the Arts** and the **Ontario Arts Council** for our publishing
program. We also acknowledge the financial support of the **Government of Canada** through the **Canada Book Fund**
and **Livres Canada Books**, and the **Government of Ontario** through the **Ontario Book Publishing Tax Credit** and the
Ontario Media Development Corporation.

Visit us at
Dundurn.com | @dundurnpress | Facebook.com/dundurnpress | Pinterest.com/Dundurnpress

Dundurn
3 Church Street, Suite 500
Toronto, Ontario, Canada
M5E 1M2

I dedicate this book to Johanne, who has always been by my side,
and to Guillaume, my steadfast companion.
To my parents for all the love they gave me.
To Catherine and Christine for their invaluable advice.

Thank you to all my friends for the evenings of wining and dining.
Thank you to all the employees and enthusiastic students at the Douglas Institute's
Centre for Study and Treatment of Circadian Rhythms.

Table of Contents

FOREWORD 11

INTRODUCTION 13

CHAPTER 1: Hitting the Sack — *Why, How, When, and Where Do We Sleep?* 17
    What is Sleep? 21
    In the Depths of Slumber 21
    Why Do We Sleep? 27
    The Neurological Mechanisms of Sleep 33
    Ways of Recording Sleep 33

CHAPTER 2: My Planet Earth — *The Biological Clock and its Rhythms* 41
    Synchronizing Our Inner and Outer Worlds 42
    Body Temperature 42
    Melatonin 44
    Cortisol 44
    Shedding Light on Our Body Clock 46
    The Other Body Clock Synchronizers 46
    The Two Processes Regulating the Sleep-Wake Cycle 50
    Circadian Rhythm Disorders 50

Night Work and Shift Work 53
Jet Lag 54
Sleep Schedule Disorders 55

CHAPTER 3: Searching for the Fountain of Youth — *Sleep at All Ages* 59
Infants 59
Children 61
Adolescents 62
Young Adults 64
Men Compared to Women 64
Mature Adults 66
The Elderly 67
Sleep and Alzheimer's Disease 68

CHAPTER 4: When You Miss the Boat — *Insomnia and You* 73
What is Insomnia? 73
What Causes Insomnia? 74
How Can You Tell How Serious Your Insomnia Is? 74
Predisposing Factors for Insomnia 77
Insomnia's Long-Term Impacts 79
Advice for Sleeping Well 81
How Can You Cure Your Insomnia? 84

CHAPTER 5: They Who Sleep Forget Their Hunger! — *Sleep and Diet* 89
Sleep and Brain Recovery 89
Sleep and Physical Recovery 91
Sleep, Body Temperature, and Energy Conservation 92

The Digestive System During the Sleep-Wake Cycle **94**
Sleep and Diet **96**
Sleep Restriction and Metabolic Disorders **97**

CHAPTER 6: Waiting For Prince Charming — *Sleeping, Waking, Light, and Mood* **101**
The Biological Clock Influences Mood **101**
The Effect of Light on Mood **102**
When Seasonal Depression Strikes **102**
Getting Into a Good Mood **105**
Depression and Sleep **107**
Bipolar Affective Disorder **109**
Premenstrual Dysphoric Disorder **112**
Anxiety **113**
Schizophrenia **113**

CHAPTER 7: The Sleeping Beauty — *Nodding Off When You Shouldn't* **117**
Narcolepsy **117**
Idiopathic Hypersomnia **127**
Secondary Daytime Sleepiness **129**
Periodic Hypersomnia **130**

CHAPTER 8: An Unexpected Climb Up Mount Everest — *Sleep Apneas* **133**
The Control of Respiration **134**
Respiration During the Sleep-Wake Cycle **136**
Sleeping at High Altitude **137**
Snoring **138**
Sleep Apnea and Sleep Hypopnea Syndrome **140**

CHAPTER 9: Bedtime Stories — *Nighttime Restlessness Disorders* 149
    Parasomnias 149
    Sleep Myoclonus 150
    Sleep-Talking 150
    Sleepwalking 150
    Night Terrors 155
    REM Sleep Behaviour Disorder 156
    Nocturnal Epilepsy 158
    Restless Legs Syndrome and Periodic Leg Movements During Sleep 160

CONCLUSION 164

ABOUT THE AUTHOR 166

TO LEARN MORE 168

IMAGE CREDITS 173

Foreword

Sleep is a part of everyday life and the subject of familiar expressions — "Good night," "Did you sleep well?" — but it's also a topic we are asking ourselves more and more questions about. Long a little-explored frontier of the neurosciences, our understanding of the mechanisms that control sleep has made remarkable strides in recent decades. Paradoxically, in the same period, a relatively new behaviour pattern has become widespread in industrialized societies: partial sleep deprivation that, day after day, lets us work longer hours, stay up later to amuse ourselves, and increases the time we spend on activities, right to the limit of what is tolerable. Thanks to artificial light, modern man has gradually developed this uniquely human behaviour pattern: no other mammal chronically deprives itself of sleep. Yet while this behaviour pattern is abnormal in terms of our biology, it is still often admired and

envied! Nonetheless, fatigue, difficulties in concentrating, the feeling of being inefficient and in a bad mood — the price paid by many for hours stolen from sleep — make us wonder: Is a manager who boasts about only getting four or five hours of sleep a night a hero or a fool?

To shed light on this complex and fascinating subject, Diane B. Boivin has written a rigorous book dealing with ideas on the cutting edge of current neurological and chronobiological research. In it she explains, in a clear and easily understandable way, why quality sleep is essential for good mental and physical health.

Many years ago, I tried to persuade Diane to come and work in my laboratory at the University of Chicago. In the end, she chose Harvard, where she made her way flawlessly through a highly charged environment, followed by a brilliant career at McGill University. The invitation to write the foreword to her first book written for the general public stems from years of respect, admiration, and friendly collegiality. It gives me the opportunity to briefly touch on my "pet subject" — the interactions between endemic sleep debt and the obesity and diabetes epidemics.

Since we sleep less and less, it's becoming more and more important to understand just how disastrous the consequences of inadequate or poor-quality sleep can be. My laboratory has been focusing on this subject for nearly fifteen years. Our initial results have encouraged other teams to explore the close connections between sleep, hormonal regulation, and cardio-metabolic risk. It's now well established that insufficient sleep has harmful effects on the hormones involved in appetite control. Limiting sleep time to four or five hours for less than a week leads to an appreciable increase in resistance to insulin, a hormone that is key to regulating glucose and lipids.

Short sleepers do exist and are described as people who manage to function reasonably well, both biologically and psychologically, on six hours a night or less, night after night. But these individuals appear to represent less than 10 percent of the population. In reality, many people who say they are short sleepers need more sleep than they think they do. The overall message of more than a hundred studies is that most adults need at least seven hours of sleep to stay biologically and psychologically healthy.

Perhaps in twenty years' time improvements in our understanding of sleep will have helped change people's perceptions, making them see that sleep is as important as proper nutrition and exercise and that it's essential to give it the attention it deserves. This book makes a major contribution and is well documented using the most up-to-date sources. The author's straightforward and lively style makes it a delight to read — and I guarantee it will keep you awake!

Thank you, Diane!

Ève Van Cauter, Ph.D.
Frederick H. Rawson Professor
Sleep, Metabolism and Health Center
The University of Chicago

What Happens in the Bedroom?

Movement is the very essence of life. I love the seasons — snow falling, melting, and falling again, the alternation of day and night and, of course, waking and sleeping. The sleep-wake cycle has always intrigued me; it is, after all, one of our body's fundamental rhythms, just like our heartbeat or breathing. When I think about this rhythm and ways to keep it steady and strong into old age, I find myself dreaming once more of the mythical Fountain of Youth ... A scientist's whimsical thoughts aside, sleep is still a fascinating state, full of mysteries and surprises. This book, not unlike deep-sea diving, is an exploratory journey into the depths of sleep. I'm offering myself as your guide on what is nothing less than a journey through its reefs! Then, when the great white shark of frustrating sleepless nights pounces on you, even though you may have to face it alone, you will have a better idea of how to fend it off.

Chapter 1 describes what sleep is, what it consists of, and how it's studied. The brain works differently depending on whether it's asleep or awake. The logic governing sleepers' behaviour is very different from the logic in control when they are awake. Activities performed when you are awake will influence the regions of the brain calling for more rest. Thus, your waking state has an effect on your sleep. Both are part of a sleep-wake cycle and are influenced by a biological clock located deep in the centre of the brain. Chapter 2 describes the biological rhythms called circadian rhythms and the disruptions that affect them. Sleep, in turn, influences your waking state. In fact, sleeping is essential if you want to be wide awake and function properly the next day. The older you get, the more you will appreciate the benefits of sleep and the impact of missing a few hours. Changes in sleep throughout life are discussed in Chapter 3, where we'll see that sleeping well helps us age better. Chapter 4 is devoted to insomnia. It describes the causes and offers advice to ease the burden.

A lack of sleep causes us to eat during the night, and sleep is closely related to diet, metabolism, and weight control. The saying "they who sleep forget their hunger" is true: this is the subject of Chapter 5. Establishing good sleep hygiene is beneficial for both physical and mental health. Chapter 6 describes sleep disturbances in various psychiatric and psychological disorders, including depression. A tendency to sleep that's too strong and extends into our periods of activity is known as daytime sleepiness. Chapter 7 deals with this subject and its clinical management in patients suffering from it. Nighttime breathing problems, largely responsible for daytime sleepiness, are the subject of Chapter 8. And sometimes the line between sleeping and waking is so fine that the two become confused in a borderline state of consciousness. Chapter 9 describes restless sleep disorders typical of such states, as well as motor problems during sleep.

This book is intended to be both an overview of the latest discoveries about sleep and a guide to help you sleep better. The hectic rhythm of modern life often — too often for some (including the author) — leads us to burn the candle at both ends. We learn very young to "live on credit" by borrowing, day after day, a few hours a week from the gods of slumber. At first glance, this reserve of hours seems to be unlimited, even free, and, because we are young, we tolerate fewer hours of sleep without experiencing repercussions on our performance in school or in our social life that are too severe. Or at least, so we think! I hope that reading this book will convince you of the opposite and of the benefits of sleep, but especially that it will provide you with useful advice. A solid understanding of what sleep and waking are and what plays a role in disrupting them is crucial. Remember that the source of the Fountain of Youth is a spring at the foot of the tree of knowledge. And just like the water from that spring, sleep too has powers of regeneration.

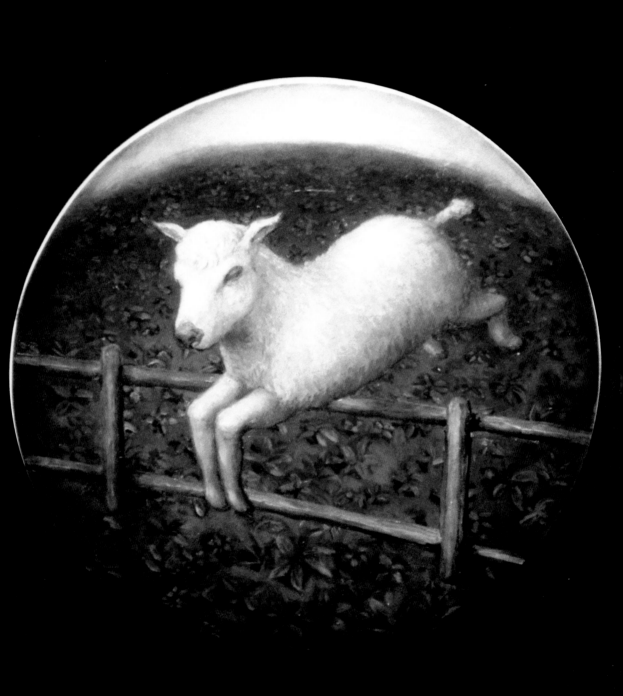

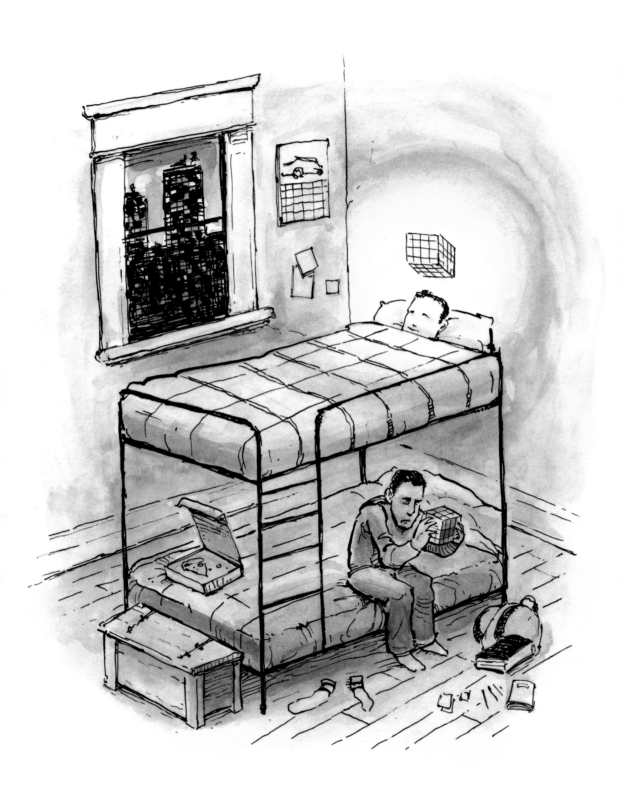

"Sleep on it" is good advice ... if you actually do sleep.

CHAPTER 1

Hitting the Sack

Why, How, When, and Where Do We Sleep?

We all know that sleep is an imperative need for each of us every day. We spend about one-third of our lives sleeping, more than the time spend working and much more than the time spend feeding ourselves. Furthermore, it's much harder not to sleep than it is not to eat. Have you ever heard of a sleep strike as a pressure tactic to support a political cause? To the author's knowledge, only one such case has been described. On the other hand, you could cite numerous examples widely covered in the media of individuals who have defended their cause with a hunger strike.

Sleep deprivation may not be very popular with activists, but torturers still find it appealing. It's on the list of methods of torture for prisoners of every stripe, and has been so for a very long time.

Sleeping is a universal need: all animals actually sleep at some point during the day. Sleep behaviours, however, vary from one species to another and from one individual to another within the same species. Human beings are no exception, and one person's sleep will certainly differ from that of another. Individual characteristics, personality traits, and lifestyles are factors affecting the length and quality of people's sleep. Sex and age are foremost among these factors. A 2005 Statistics Canada survey (all ages combined) shows that men sleep for approximately eight hours and seven minutes daily, or eleven minutes less than women (Figure 1). This is a surprising observation, for we know that women have more trouble sleeping than men do. Researchers have not yet solved this mystery. Sleep quality, however, tends to deteriorate more as we age. Once people reach their forties or fifties, most are more easily awakened during the night, even if they slept like a baby in their twenties. This alone makes them more susceptible to insomnia. But beware — aging begins long before we get our senior citizen's card! In terms of sleep, we're already past our prime when we blow out thirty-five candles ...

Our activities also affect our sleep, and first among these is work, which still occupies a very large portion of our lives. People who are workaholics and those who feel they don't have enough time seem to sleep twenty-one and twenty-nine minutes less per day, respectively, than people less preoccupied by their work or by time. If people who lack time work five days a week and forty-eight weeks a year, they therefore sleep roughly 116 hours less than less harried workers. It isn't surprising that workaholics sleep less, since they borrow time from where they think they have extra — their sleep. Their annual sleep debt is probably much higher than the above figures indicate, and over time this can have undesirable consequences. One interesting fact is that sleep time tends to decrease as annual income climbs (Figure 2). This doesn't mean you have to "work for peanuts" to sleep well, but it would be good to give sleep the credit it deserves. It's better not to dismiss it out of hand, unthinkingly, when we believe we have more important things to do, because we might wake up one day and realize it was our best ally. People who take more than an hour to get to the office and those who work full time lose on average twenty-two and twenty minutes of sleep a day, respectively, compared to those who live closer to their work or don't work. So, if you live in the suburbs and work downtown, don't forget to add the human cost (sleep debt) to the economic cost (gas, faster wear and tear on your car) in your budget!

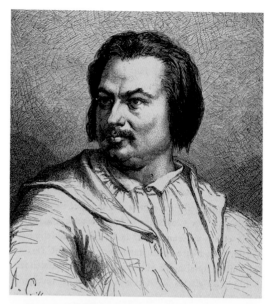

Sleep Little, Sleep a Lot

"There is no sorrow that sleep cannot overcome."

HONORÉ DE BALZAC
(TRANS. ELLEN MARRIAGE)
Cousin Pons

Barely one in seven persons is a healthy short or long sleeper who sleeps fewer than six hours or more than nine hours a night.* Albert Einstein, a physicist, slept from ten to eleven hours a night, in order, he said, to nurture the creative process. Five hours' sleep was more than enough for Winston Churchill, and Napoleon Bonaparte claimed he only needed four hours a night. And Balzac, who, judging by this quote, appeared to value the benefits of good quality sleep, in fact lived completely differently: a writer whose work habits are legendary, he drank as many as thirty cups of coffee a day so as to remain awake and work through the night.

* S. E. Luckhaupt et al., 2010.

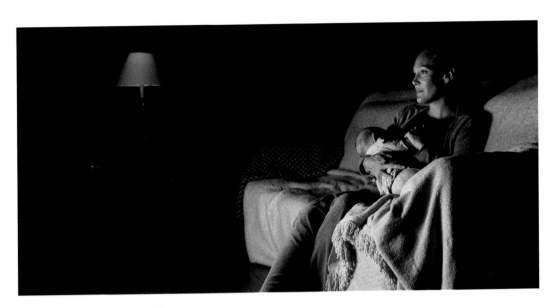

AVERAGE SLEEP TIME*

	Men Average : 487 min.	Women Average : 498 min.
HOW OLD ARE YOU?		
15 to 24	517 min.	527 min.
25 to 39	483 min.	487 min.
40 to 59	472 min.	487 min.**
60 and over	491 min.	508 min.**
WHAT IS YOUR MARITAL STATUS?		
Single	506 min.	513 min.
Married or common law	478 min.	493 min.**
Separated or divorced	485 min.	484 min.
Widowed	487 min.	506 min.
DO YOU HAVE CHILDREN UNDER 15?		
No	491 min.	503 min.**
1	476 min.	486 min.
2 or more	466 min.	478 min.
DO YOU ALWAYS FEEL STRESSED?		
No	493 min.	505 min.**
Yes	472 min.	487 min.**
DO YOU FEEL YOU DON'T HAVE ENOUGH TIME?		
Seldom	499 min.	511 min.**
Sometimes	485 min.	494 min.**
Often	464 min.	486 min.**

* 8 hours of sleep equals 480 min.
** Significantly different values for men and women.

FIGURE 1   Statistics Canada, *General Social Survey*, 2005.

AVERAGE SLEEP TIME AND WORK*

	Men	Women
DO YOU THINK OF YOURSELF AS A WORKAHOLIC?		
No	493 min.	503 min.*
Yes	470 min.	484 min.**
WHAT IS YOUR WORK STATUS?		
None	503 min.	505 min.
Part-time	491 min.	493 min.
Full-time	474 min.	488 min.**
WHAT IS YOUR WORK SCHEDULE?		
Daytime work	474 min.	488 min.**
Other schedules	482 min.	495 min.
HOW LONG DOES IT TAKE YOU TO GET TO WORK?		
1 to 30 min.	475 min.	491 min.**
31 to 60 min.	472 min.	482 min.
60 min. or more	451 min.	474 min.**
WHAT IS YOUR ANNUAL INCOME?		
$0 to $19,999	509 min.	510 min.
$20,000 to $39,999	484 min.	485 min.
$40,000 to $59,999	472 min.	476 min.
$60,000 and over	466 min.	479 min.

*8 hours of sleep equals 480 min.
** Significantly different values for men and women.

FIGURE 2

Statistics Canada, *General Social Survey*, 2005.

Given the frantic pace typical of modern life, it's not surprising that we should try to recover some sleep on our days off. We sleep more on Saturdays and Sundays, getting out of bed on average an hour later than on weekday mornings. But as we might have expected, family responsibilities are also major sleep thieves. For example, parents with two or more children under fifteen years of age sleep twenty-five minutes less each day than childless adults. Not counting the period after birth, having children and looking after them means sacrificing nearly 148 hours of sleep per year!

So why do we have to sleep so much when it seems there are so many better things to do?

WHAT IS SLEEP?

Sleep is a phase of relaxation and recovery that follows a waking period during which an individual accumulates a sleep debt. During sleep, sleepers are less aware of their environment, but this is a rapidly reversible state, since people can be awakened by a noise or a jolt. This makes sleep different from a loss of consciousness or a comatose state from which an individual cannot be immediately awakened. The behaviours adopted during sleep are peculiar to the sleeping person or animal. An interesting comparison can be made of sleep positions and the amount of sleep required in different animal species (Figure 3).

IN THE DEPTHS OF SLUMBER

To fully understand sleep and its disorders, it's important to know how sleep is structured throughout the night. In fact, sleep is a very complex state made up of several distinct phases called sleep stages. These stages are divided into cycles lasting about ninety minutes each and occurring one after another during the night. The period between going to sleep in the evening and waking up in the morning is called a sleep episode. Let's look more closely at these sleep stages and the way they are organized in cycles during a nighttime sleep episode.

The various states of vigilance are called sleep stages. These fall into two main categories, REM (rapid eye movement) sleep, also called paradoxical sleep, and non-REM sleep. Non-REM sleep consists of stages 1 and 2, both stages of lighter sleep, as well as slow wave sleep, consisting of stages 3 and 4. An average night is made up of roughly 25 percent REM sleep and 75 percent non-REM sleep. As well, sleep is interrupted many times during the night; sleepers are usually not aware of these awakenings because they last such a short time. For purposes of comparison, it's useful to begin describing the stages of sleep by describing what it means to be awake.

Wakefulness is the main state of consciousness, normally lasting from sixteen to seventeen hours each day. The rest of the day, seven to eight hours, is for sleeping. As we have indicated, sleep also contains periods of wakefulness. Approximately 10 percent of our sleep periods are actually spent in a waking state. These intermittent periods of wakefulness

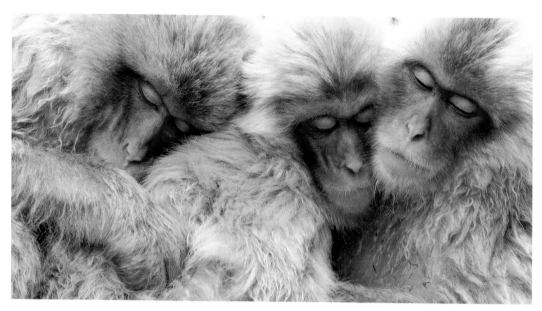

HOW DO ANIMALS SLEEP?

Animal*	Position**	Length and time of sleep
Giraffe	• Lying on the ground, head resting on its hind legs and neck arched	• In short naps lasting 2½ to 6 min. • Approximately 4½ hours/day • At night
Elephant	• Lying on its side on the ground	• 1 to 4½ hours/day • At night
Koala	• Sitting on a tree branch	• 16 to 18 hours/day • Day and night
Horse	• Standing or lying down	• In short naps • Approximately 2½ hours/day • At night
Cat	• Lying on its stomach or rolled into a ball	• Up to 16 hours/day • Day and night
Lion	• Lying on its stomach on the ground	• Up to 20 hours/day when hunting • Day and night
Bat	• Hanging by its feet on a cave wall	• Up to 20 hours/day • In the daytime
Rat	• Lying on its stomach	• Approximately 10 hours/day • In the daytime

* There are differences among individuals of the same species, owing to their genetic baggage.
** Other sleep positions can be seen.

FIGURE 3

Adapted from *www.scienceblogs.com*, *www.animal.discovery.com*.

enable sleepers to change position and be alert to their environment from time to time during the night. It's even probable that these spontaneous awakenings were an advantage for the survival of the species in our Stone Age ancestors. Wakefulness is recognized by the high level of brain activity it involves; in these periods, an electroencephalogram (EEG) shows a variety of low-amplitude, high-frequency waves. These high-frequency waves indicate that several regions of the brain are simultaneously activated, since the brain is bombarded with information from all sides, information it then analyzes and acts on. When a person is on the verge of falling asleep, the brain gradually relaxes; so-called alpha waves are then frequently observed in the posterior occipital regions of the brain. This state of calm wakefulness is conducive to falling asleep.

During stage 1 sleep, brain activity slows down, muscle tone remains high, the eyes roll slightly, and the sleeper is easily awakened. This stage lasts from one to seven minutes in a young sleeper. Since stage 1 sleep is so light, the sleeper has the impression of being between two worlds, neither asleep nor awake. Some people awakened during stage 1 will swear with conviction that they haven't slept. This stage occupies about 10 percent of a sleep episode.

In stage 2 sleep, distinctive graphic elements appear on the electroencephalogram sleep spindles and K-complexes. The appearance of these elements on the recording is important, as it indicates beyond any doubt that sleep is well and truly established. In fact, these graphic signs of sleep show that communication circuits between the deep and superficial

The Sleep Strike as a Pressure Tactic

In 2009 a union local in an electronics company in Fréha, in the Algerian territorial community of Tizi Ouzou, was forced to use various pressure tactics. In addition to one-hour demonstrations inside the company, sit-ins outside management's offices, and hunger strikes, its workers tried a completely new tactic: a sleep strike. Having challenged themselves to stay awake together until their demands were satisfied, nine unionists went without sleep for ten days. In the end they won, but the consequences of their action on their health are unknown.

BRAIN ACTIVITY DURING SLEEP

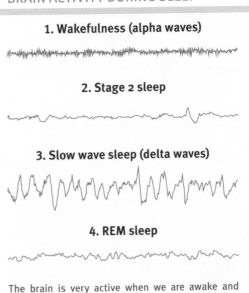

1. Wakefulness (alpha waves)

2. Stage 2 sleep

3. Slow wave sleep (delta waves)

4. REM sleep

The brain is very active when we are awake and during REM sleep. It slows down during stage 2 sleep and is at its least active during slow wave sleep.

FIGURE 4   EEG readings from Dr. D.B. Boivin's laboratory.

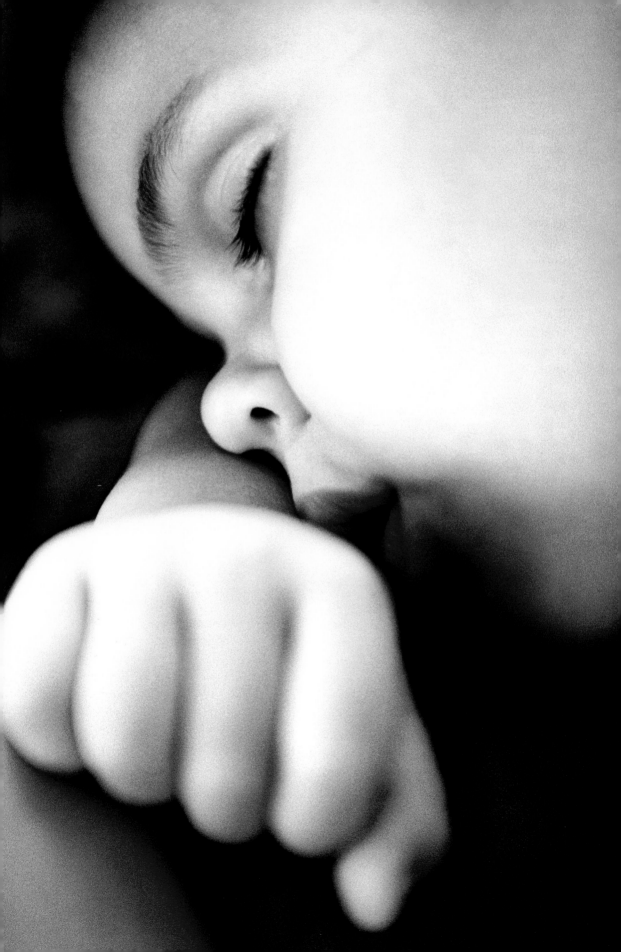

regions of the brain, called thalamo-cortical loops, are functioning. These loops signal that the process of "disconnecting" the brain from its environment has begun and that the brain has started its recovery work, with the goal of eliminating the neuronal fatigue accumulated during the day. Stage 2 is considered to be the very basis of sleep, accounting for 40 to 50 percent of a night's sleep. There is a stronger perception of having slept, compared with stage 1, meaning that sleepers will agree that they have slept, if awakened from stage 2 sleep.

Slow wave sleep begins thirty to forty-five minutes after we fall asleep. The arousal threshold is higher than in stage 1 or 2 sleep, and the brain is in a deep resting phase. At this point, a healthy sleeper is calm and deeply asleep and the electroencephalogram reading shows high-amplitude slow delta waves. These waves indicate that several parts of the brain are resting at the same time and are synchronized among themselves. This sleep is often subdivided into stage 3 and 4 sleep, depending on the proportion of time when delta waves are present. When 20 to 50 percent of the EEG reading is composed of delta waves, it's referred to as stage 3, as compared to stage 4, where delta waves are in the majority. Sleepers are harder to wake up from slow wave sleep than from the lighter stages 1 and 2 sleep. What's more, someone who is forced to wake up out of slow wave sleep will take much longer to become fully alert than if they had been awakened from a stage of lighter sleep. This is what happens when the telephone rings or the baby cries when we are sleeping soundly and it takes us some time to wake up. Known as sleep inertia (see Chapter 9), this condition can be problematic for professionals on call who have to make important decisions during the night.

Sleep Deprivation as a Torture Device

Sleep deprivation is a useful therapeutic tool and has beneficial effects when used to treat patients with depression. However, depriving human beings of sleep is also among the most "effective" means of torturing them. Victims are forced to stand and when they look likely to fall asleep, this is physically prevented by subjecting them to loud or grating noises and bright light. The procedure is repeated for between 48 and 180 hours, or up to more than a week without sleep, to obtain the desired results. Among other things, victims experience hallucinations, confusion, and memory lapses; they develop headaches, cognitive deficits, elevated stress hormone and blood pressure levels, and muscle soreness.

All over the world, many political prisoners and prisoners of war have been deprived of sleep to extract information from them or humiliate them. Used by the former Soviet Union and various totalitarian regimes and by national security services, as well as in the American prison at Guantanamo, sleep deprivation is one of the methods of torture condemned by the UN and by Amnesty International.

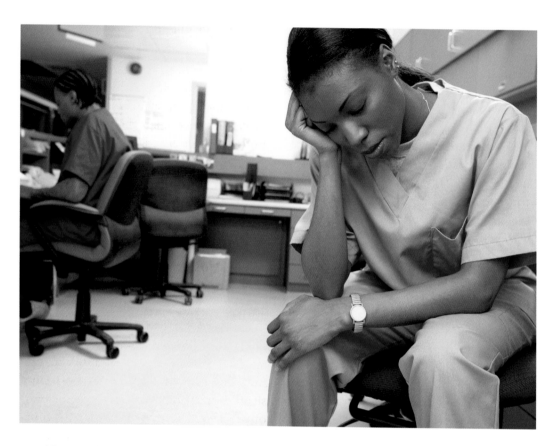

About 25 percent of a sleep episode consists of slow wave sleep. This is a very important phase, as it is largely in this stage that our brain recovers from fatigue accumulated the day before.

Approximately seventy to one hundred minutes after falling asleep, a very distinctive stage of sleep, called REM sleep, begins. It is unusual in that it has characteristics of both sleep and wakefulness. On one hand, the arousal threshold is very high in this stage and the sleeper is deeply asleep. On the other, the brain is very active and brain activity resembles the activity of the waking state much more than that of other sleep stages. The curious combination of a very active brain and a state of deep sleep has earned it the name of paradoxical sleep. The onset of this stage is marked by three specific phenomena that occur at the same time. First, the brain is very active, almost as active as when it's awake. Secondly, sleepers experience rapid eye movements. Lastly, sleepers are temporarily paralysed. Indeed, the tone of their skeletal muscles — those important for maintaining posture and arm and leg function — drops drastically. Paralysis occurs periodically during the night in healthy sleepers, in the periods of REM sleep. Other physiological changes also occur: a rapid and irregular pulse, erratic breathing, constricted pupils, muscle spasms, and nocturnal erections. During REM sleep, body temperature control is disrupted, causing sleepers to become sensitive to bedroom temperature fluctuations. This state is often compared to that observed in cold-blooded animals like reptiles. We thus go back to our "reptilian state" briefly every night, approximately every ninety minutes. An interesting fact is that REM sleep is the stage in which we dream.

These stages of sleep occur in sequence and are repeated several times during the night. They are organized into cycles of roughly ninety to one hundred minutes each. As a rule, sleep cycles begin and end with periods of REM sleep. We therefore experience periods of REM sleep and, as a result, dreams, about every ninety minutes. Even healthy people who think they never dream actually do so four to six times a night. It's just that they don't remember. The kind of sleep in each cycle also varies during the night. The first cycles include a great deal of slow wave sleep, whereas the last cycles contain more REM sleep. Slow wave sleep therefore predominates in the early part of the night, while REM sleep shows the opposite pattern. This is explained by the fact that the first hours of the night are primarily when we recover from accumulated fatigue, while the last hours of rest are when we dream.

WHY DO WE SLEEP?

You spend a lot of time sleeping, without being too sure why. Well, this apparently very simple question about the purpose of sleep is more complex than it first appears. Even today, we are still waiting for a definitive answer to this question. With this goal in mind, researchers have studied the consequences of sleep deprivation (Van Dongen et al., 2004). Sleep deprivation may be total (forced wakefulness all night long) or partial (a period of sleep cut short). It can also be restricted to a specific sleep stage, as in REM sleep deprivation, for example. By studying what happens in individuals deprived of sleep, we can begin to better understand why we sleep.

With this question as a backdrop, American researchers carried out extreme sleep deprivation experiments at the end of the 1960s. In these experiments, four volunteers were kept awake for 205 hours in a row, or more than eight days (Pasnau et al., 1968; Kollar et al., 1969). A gradual increase in fatigue and a decline in mental abilities and psychometric performance were observed. Intermittent personality

What Happens in Bed?

It's normal to change position several times during sleep. In medical parlance, the reclining position is called decubitus. Positions taken during sleep have been given several names, depending on whether a person is lying on his or her back (dorsal decubitus), front (ventral decubitus), left side (left lateral decubitus), or right side (right lateral decubitus). To make the time you spend in bed as restful as possible, you must have good sleep hygiene. This means cultivating positive lifestyle habits that encourage sufficient recovery at night and high levels of vigilance the next day. A review of sleep hygiene is an integral part of treating almost all sleep disorders. Several pieces of advice for improving sleep hygiene will be given throughout this book.

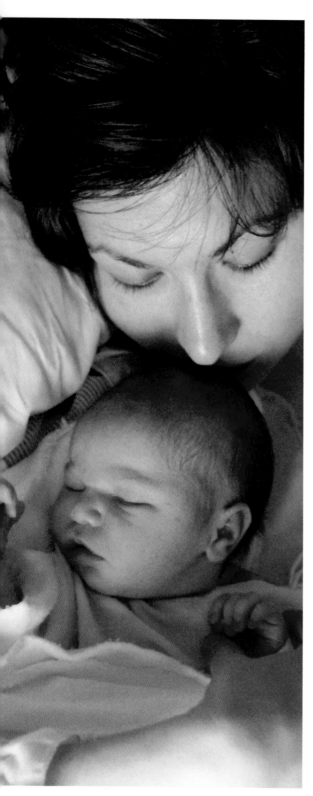

disorders appeared — irritability, immature behaviour, sensory distortions, and hallucinations. On the third day, participants were unable to read because they couldn't concentrate. As the hours of wakefulness accumulated, the participants' brain activity changed, taken over by slow delta waves that normally occur in slow wave sleep. These young men behaved as though they had been woken up, when in reality their brains were both awake and asleep. They lost the thread of events over and over again, and often lacked muscle tone to the point of nearly falling down.

These mixed states between sleeping and waking indicate that the border between these two worlds is not always well guarded. Working in conditions that require prolonged wakefulness is obviously dangerous, especially if a person has to drive a vehicle, use weapons, or operate heavy equipment. When work is unrelenting and compulsory, some individuals may be tempted to use psychostimulants to help them stay awake more easily. Unfortunately, doing so can have disastrous consequences. Sleep remains a necessity and it will try to have its way no matter what, even if we try to prevent it. It will even worm its way into our waking process if it has to. In some patients, the line between waking and sleeping is so fine and so permeable that the two states occur simultaneously, their characteristics intermingling in a state of borderline consciousness when they should be separate. This unusual and fascinating type of sleep disorder will be described in Chapter 9.

Sleeping at night is therefore essential if we want to be wide awake and alert the next day. When we allow our sleep to suffer, our waking time suffers as well. This

THE STAGES OF SLEEP

State	Description	Brain activity (measured on an EEG)	Other phenomena (measured on an EMG or EOG)
Wakefulness	Individuals respond to their environment. Many awakenings also occur during normal sleep.	Several regions of the brain are activated simultaneously. An active brain shows rapid low-amplitude waves. In a relaxed individual, alpha waves (8–13 Hz*) can be seen on an EEG of the posterior regions of the skull.	• High muscle tone corresponding to the individual's physical activity. • Eyes move in the direction the person is looking.
Stage 1 sleep (recently renamed N1 sleep)	Light sleep and the sensation of being "between two worlds." Sleepers are easy to wake up.	Slowdown in brain activity on an EEG. The speed of the waves decreases and slightly slower waves called theta waves (4–7 Hz) begin to appear.	• Muscle tone weaker than when awake, but still high. • Eyes roll slowly.
Stage 2 (recently renamed N2 sleep)	This stage is the basis of sleep. Sleepers are fully aware they have been sleeping.	Brain activity slows down further. On an EEG distinctive graphic elements indicating sleep begin to appear: sleep spindles (phases of activation of 12–14 Hz) and K-complexes (biphasic waves lasting at least .5 seconds).	• Muscle tone weaker than when awake, but still high. • No eye movements.
Slow wave sleep — stages 3 and 4 (recently renamed N3 sleep)	Deep sleep during which sleepers are hard to wake up. They appear confused when forced to wake up.	Brain activity is at its lowest level. The EEG is synchronized and dominated by high-amplitude slow waves, or delta waves (0.5–4 Hz). In stage 3, these waves are present 20 to 50 percent of the time. In stage 4, they dominate the EEG reading more than 50 percent of the time.	• Muscle tone weaker than when awake. • No eye movements.
REM sleep (also called paradoxical sleep)	Sleepers are sleeping deeply and dreaming intensely. Dreams are reported after 85 percent of awakenings during this stage.	The brain is almost as active as when it's awake. This surprising state — a sleeper deeply asleep, paralyzed, but with a very active brain — earned this stage the name of paradoxical sleep.	• Loss of muscle tone indicating that the sleeper is paralyzed. • Rapid eye movements (REM) visible on an EOG.

* Hz quantifies the frequency of oscillations.

FIGURE 5

Dreams and Nocturnal Erections

REM sleep is the stage associated with dreams, so much so that when awakened from this stage, sleepers will report having dreamed in 85 percent of cases, compared with 15 percent when they wake up out of another stage of sleep. In 1929 Sigmund Freud published a book titled *Die Traumdeutung (The Interpretation of Dreams)*. The fact that this book was published attests to the interest the medical community of the time had in the contents of dreams as a tool for understanding the causes of psychological and psychiatric disorders. The occurrence of nocturnal erections during REM sleep led some researchers to examine the erotic content of dreams in an attempt to explain these phenomena. To the Freudians' great regret, there is no connection between nocturnal erections and the contents of dreams. They are a purely physiological phenomenon. Research into the unconscious will have to find another route.

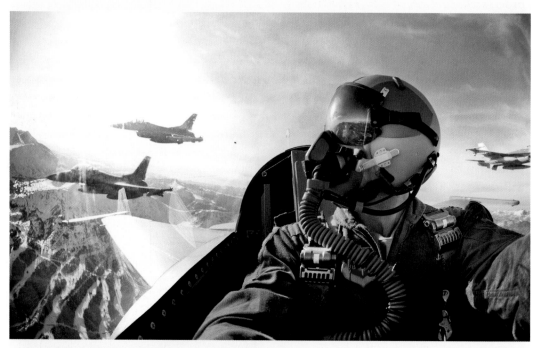

Danger: A Deadly Way to Stay Awake

Who can forget the tragic accident in Afghanistan in April 2002, when four Canadian soldiers were killed by a laser-guided bomb dropped by an American fighter jet. The American Air Force spokesperson explained at the time: "When fatigue could be expected to degrade air crew performance, they are given Dexedrine in 10 mg doses." It's still not known whether Dexedrine played a role in this accident, although this possibility has been raised by at least one military analyst.

statement is not surprising, since one of sleep's primary functions is recovery. We sleep to recover from the physical and mental fatigue accumulated during the day. It follows that the more tired we are, the greater our need for sleep. This can be compared to a debt that starts to build up the minute we put our big toe out of bed, and even, to be more precise, as soon as we open our eyes. Many studies have validated this so-called homeostatic function of sleep and shown that the pressure — the need for sleep — increases in proportion to how long we have been awake. This process can be explained by using an hourglass in which the grains of sand begin to flow into one of the bulbs when we get up and flow out when we go to bed, when we turn the hourglass over. Thus, the longer we are awake, the more grains of sand accumulate in the bulb of the hourglass and the more our need for sleep increases. It will also take more time to empty the sand that has accumulated, meaning we will have to sleep longer. Scientists often compare delta waves to grains of sand (Borbély et al., 1999). It's primarily at the beginning of the night during slow wave sleep, with its high concentration of delta waves, that we pay back our sleep debt. This should be reassuring — our brain has understood that it has to pay back its sleep debt before it starts to dream.

We may wonder what all these stages of sleep are for. Scientists have tried depriving sleepers of certain specific stages to see what would happen. Conducting these experiments — known as studies of the selective deprivation of sleep stages — often requires considerable, not to say heroic, efforts, as they require intensive monitoring of research participants all

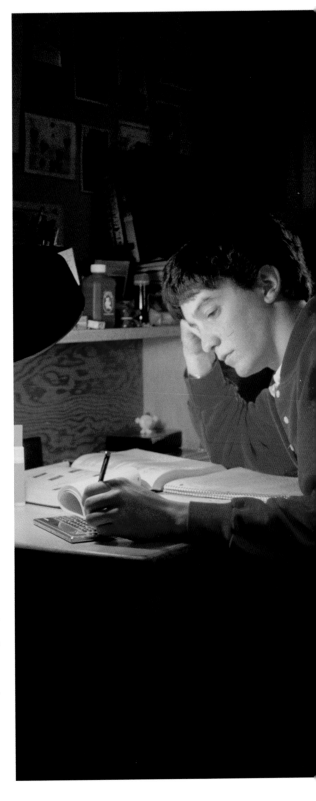

Sleep, Learning, and Memory

Acquiring new knowledge requires an initial encoding of sensory and motor experiences. A subsequent process is necessary to consolidate this initially fragile knowledge and store it as lasting memories. There are several indications that sleep plays an important role in learning by enhancing brain plasticity. While we sleep, processes come into play that allow new knowledge to be organized and help turn it into long-term memories. During sleep, new knowledge travels along a kind of assembly line, at the end of which it's stored as lasting knowledge.

Learning is therefore reinforced after a good night's sleep, compared with a night of sleep deprivation. The first night after the day of learning seems to be the most important, although the process of organizing new knowledge can continue for several months. A word to students who cram all night, at the last minute, for an exam: those intense efforts will be a poor long-term investment compared with a few study sessions followed by good nights of sleep.

The benefits of sleep also apply to learning new complex motor skills, like how to play a new sport or musical instrument. Athletes know that if physical workouts are too frequent and intense, their performance will decline. Planning a nap of sixty minutes or more can prevent this and enhance performance, even without further practice. What's more, the amount of REM sleep and stage 2 sleep tends to increase the night after new techniques have been learned. Athletes in training will thus make faster progress if they sleep better.

Sleep also enables us to find creative solutions to complex problems. When young students were asked to solve a difficult mathematical problem, they found an original solution after a good night's sleep, whereas another group that had stayed up all night did not manage to solve the math problem (Wagner et al., 2004). Sleep appears to encourage new links among neuronal networks in the brain. So it's absolutely true that we should sleep on it!

night and all day, for many weeks in a row. In human beings, experiments in selective REM sleep deprivation were conducted over several weeks with depressed patients (Vogel et al., 1980). An antidepressant effect was observed in approximately one out of two patients, indicating that this stage of sleep has a significant effect on psychological health. The role of sleep in mental health will be discussed in greater depth in Chapter 6. In healthy sleepers, on the other hand, REM sleep deprivation seems to have negative effects on mood and memory consolidation.

Recent experiments have used sound stimuli to wake up subjects repeatedly during slow wave sleep (Tasali et al., 2008). These studies have shown that a reduction in slow wave sleep leads to disruptions in blood sugar metabolism. We will come back to the metabolic consequences of sleep disorders in Chapter 5.

Sleep Homeostasis

Homeostasis is a system's ability to maintain its equilibrium in spite of external disturbances, and sleep homeostasis is the ability of the sleep system to recover its equilibrium in circumstances causing sleep deprivation. Maintaining homeostasis in the physiological systems of the human body is important for keeping us alive.

THE NEUROLOGICAL MECHANISMS OF SLEEP

No single substance appears to be essential and indispensable to falling asleep and staying asleep. Instead, a multitude of substances and neuronal circuits come into play at different times of day. However, centres in the brain that are essential for sleeping and waking have been identified (Figure 8). For example, we fall asleep at bedtime when the sleep centres are activated and the wake centres calm down. The opposite happens when we get up. It's almost as though a switch was flipped to trigger the sleep function at bedtime. The switch is then reset for the waking function when it's time to wake up. There is reciprocal inhibition between the wake and sleep centres, creating an alternating sleep-wake cycle. Thus, when subjects are sleeping, their sleep centres are active. These gradually lose their strength during the night, as the wake centres get progressively stronger. The opposite occurs at bedtime. This system of transitions from sleeping to waking (and the opposite) is called the flip-flop switch or sleep-wake switch cycle (Saper et al., 2010).

WAYS OF RECORDING SLEEP

Sleep is a complex and many-faceted universe. Studying it therefore demands a sophisticated approach, involving the

A NEURON

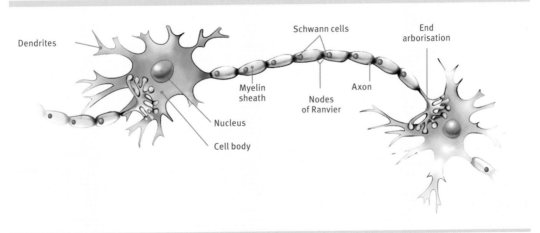

Dendrites
Schwann cells
End arborisation
Myelin sheath
Nodes of Ranvier
Axon
Nucleus
Cell body

FIGURE 6

Sleep in Animal Species

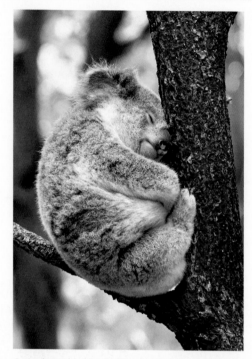

In primates, including humans, sleep is monophasic or biphasic, consisting of a main period of sleep with or without a short daytime nap. In most other mammals, sleep is polyphasic and occurs in short frequent naps either by day or by night, depending on whether the species is diurnal or nocturnal. In terms of adaptation, sleep can be a disadvantage, since the animal is less aware of its environment and becomes easier prey for its predators. This means that the daily organization of sleep and sleep behaviours are strongly influenced by a species' ecological niche. Thus, prey spend less time in REM sleep (during which they are paralyzed) than do predators. And animals that are more sensitive to temperature fluctuations in their environment, like small animals and those that live in temperate climates, have shorter sleep cycles.

An unusual kind of sleep, unihemispheric sleep, is seen in aquatic mammals like dolphins or wild ducks. What this means is that one brain hemisphere sleeps deeply while the other is awake. These periods of unihemispheric sleep last about forty minutes and alternate from one hemisphere to the other. In this state, the animal can swim to the surface to breathe while one hemisphere at a time is asleep. Since brain functions are crossed, the active contralateral hemisphere allows the other side of the body to keep functioning. For example, the active right hemisphere keeps the left eye open. Unihemispheric sleep also allows these species to swim in groups, with the animals on the periphery of the group using their open eye to look outwards, so they can react immediately to any danger, the perfect example of a social environment watch strategy (Figure 7).

Generally speaking, the total duration of sleep and slow wave sleep is inversely proportional to the size of the animal and its metabolic rate. Thus, smaller animals (in terms of both body and head) with a rapid metabolism sleep more than do large mammals with a slow metabolism. Small mammals also have greater nutritional needs and live shorter lives than large mammals. If this is so, then why does a koala sleep so much, despite being bigger and less active than a pigeon?

Koalas sleep a lot to conserve more energy, since their diet, composed mainly of eucalyptus leaves low in nutritive value, is deficient. They who sleep forget their hunger, as they say. Studies stress the importance of sleep, and in particular that of slow wave sleep, in conserving animals' energy reserves.

As for REM sleep, it seems to play a major role in brain maturation. This is why species born immature — called altricial species and including human beings — spend more time in REM sleep than precocial species, born with a mature brain. The proportion of time spent in REM sleep in the former species decreases gradually as the central nervous system matures, until it reaches the levels seen in adults.

UNHEMISPHERIC SLEEP IN A POD OF DOLPHINS

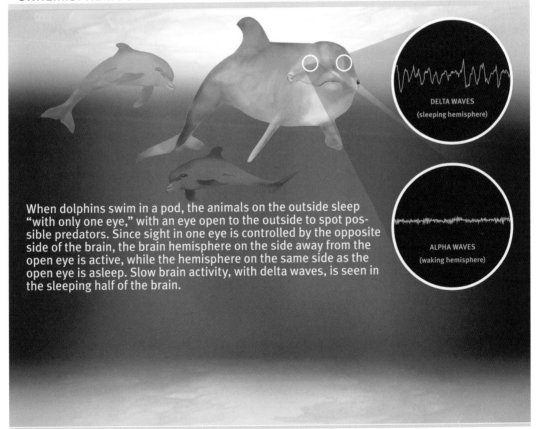

DELTA WAVES
(sleeping hemisphere)

ALPHA WAVES
(waking hemisphere)

When dolphins swim in a pod, the animals on the outside sleep "with only one eye," with an eye open to the outside to spot possible predators. Since sight in one eye is controlled by the opposite side of the brain, the brain hemisphere on the side away from the open eye is active, while the hemisphere on the same side as the open eye is asleep. Slow brain activity, with delta waves, is seen in the sleeping half of the brain.

FIGURE 7

THE SLEEP-WAKE CYCLE

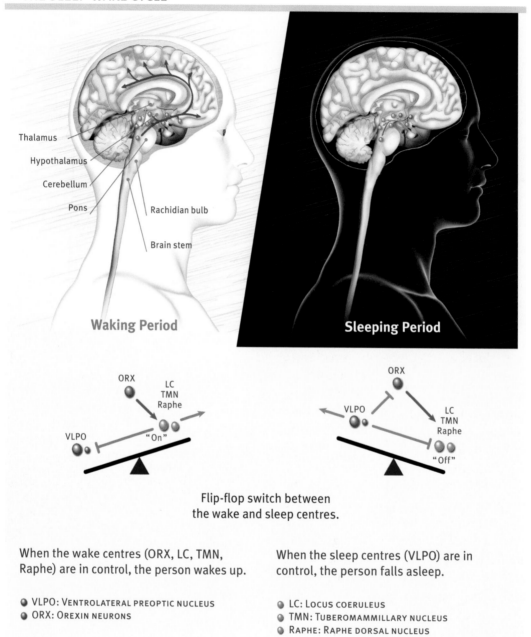

Flip-flop switch between
the wake and sleep centres.

When the wake centres (ORX, LC, TMN, Raphe) are in control, the person wakes up.

When the sleep centres (VLPO) are in control, the person falls asleep.

- VLPO: Ventrolateral preoptic nucleus
- ORX: Orexin neurons

- LC: Locus coeruleus
- TMN: Tuberomammillary nucleus
- Raphe: Raphe dorsal nucleus

FIGURE 8

Based on Saper, 2006.

recording of biological signals obtained from different regions on the sleeper's head. Electrical activity in the brain produced by neurons is recorded by attaching between six and twenty-four electrodes to the subject's scalp, from left to right and front to back. More complex set-ups, using more electrodes, are used when a neurological problem is suspected. Electrical signals from the brain are then recorded by these electrodes and transferred via conductive wires to a computer to create a signal called an electroencephalogram (EEG). This signal makes it possible to measure the waves shown in Figure 4. These waves are important in identifying sleep stages. Eye movements are also recorded as they allow us to recognize REM sleep. They are documented using electrodes placed one or two centimetres from the edge of the sleeper's eyes. Since the cornea has a positive charge, in contrast to the retina, eye movements create a current that is captured by these electrodes and transferred through a conductive wire to a computer to create a signal called an electrooculogram (EOG).

As we have seen, in REM sleep the sleeper experiences episodes of muscle paralysis. It's therefore important to measure muscle tone during the night using electrodes placed on the chin muscles. The muscular contractions responsible for the tone of these muscles also generate an electrical current, captured by these electrodes and transferred by conductive wires to a computer to create a signal called an electromyogram (EMG).

These three biological signals are necessary to identify the sleep stage the sleeper is in (Figure 5). Since several biological signals are recorded simultaneously, the

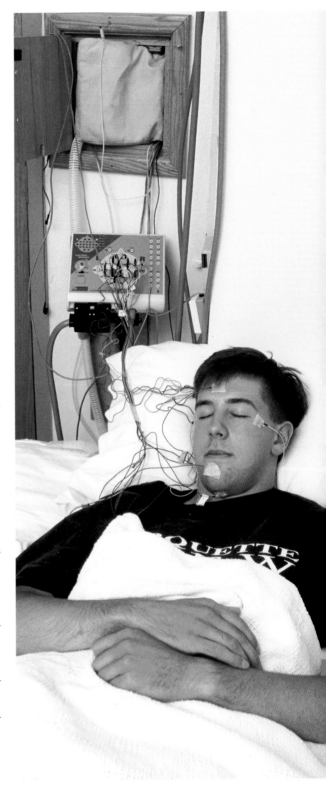

HYPNOGRAM SHOWING THE STAGES OF SLEEP

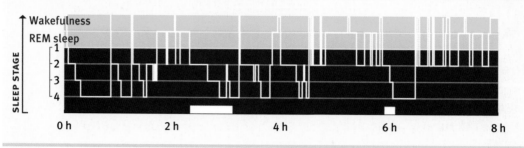

FIGURE 9   Hypnogram of a 37-year-old man, from Dr. D.B. Boivin's laboratory.

sleep recording is called a polysomno-graphic recording. This term is derived from the Greek roots *poly* ("several"), *somno* ("sleep"), and *gráphô* ("to write").

Once the sleep recording has been made, it's analyzed in very short segments of about thirty seconds each called sleep epochs. A stage of sleep is attributed to each of these epochs and the sequence of sleep stages throughout the night is illustrated using a graph called a sleep hypnogram (Figure 9). In each eight-hour-long night of sleep, 960 sleep epochs are therefore produced. Luckily, paper recordings have been replaced by digital recordings, because it used to take more than one box of neurological recording paper to document this information. Analyzing a night's sleep thus requires a lot of work. This explains in part why the wait is so long to get an appointment at a sleep clinic.

To sum up, sleep is a state of altered consciousness involving a withdrawal into our inner world and a progressively decreasing sensitivity to our environment. We therefore spend at least a third of our lives relatively disconnected from reality. During sleep, the organism goes through a series of stages, each with different levels of brain activity that promote, on the one hand, recovery from the fatigue accumulated during the day and, on the other, the integration of knowledge acquired the day before. It's therefore not surprising that this complex mechanism sometimes fails. Fully understanding what normal sleep is enables us to understand better the conditions that negatively affect its quality.

What Should You Take
Away From This Chapter?

- There are two main kinds of sleep — REM sleep (standing for rapid eye movement), sometimes called paradoxical sleep, and non-REM sleep. Non-REM sleep is itself subdivided into stages 1 and 2, and slow wave sleep (also called stages 3 and 4).

- During the night, sleep is organized into recurring cycles lasting approximately ninety minutes each. Slow wave sleep predominates in the early cycles, while REM sleep predominates in the later ones.

- Slow wave sleep and the delta brain waves that accompany it are indicative of its recovery function.

- REM sleep is traditionally associated with dreams and involves an active brain in a subject who is sleeping deeply, whose eyes are moving and whose body is paralyzed.

- Length and quality of sleep vary from person to person and according to lifestyle habits.

- Disrupted sleep also disrupts mental and physical functioning during the day. You will function better and longer if you give sleep its rightful place.

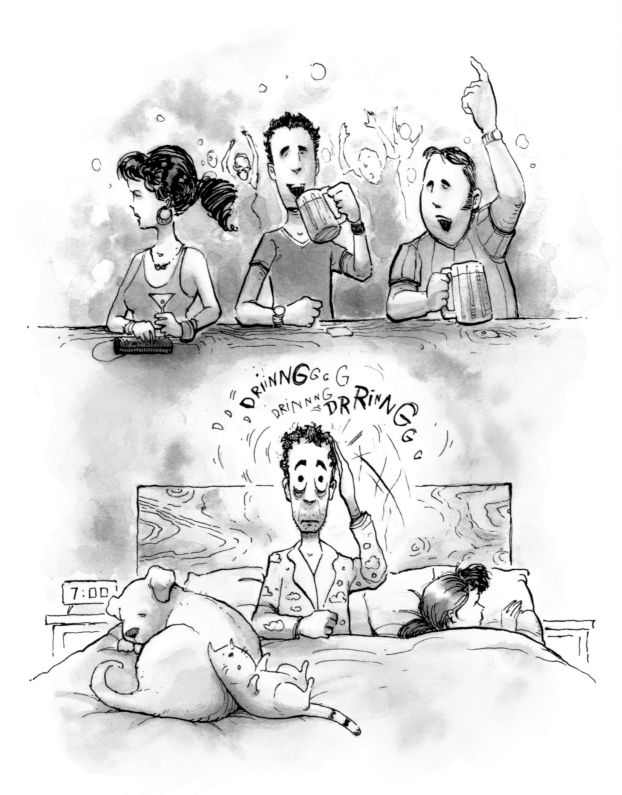

The biological clock couldn't care less about the morning after.

CHAPTER 2

My Planet Earth

The Biological Clock and its Rythms

Different animal species behave differently over the course of a day. So-called diurnal animals are more active during the day, whereas nocturnal animals are more active at night. But mixed activity habits are also seen (M. Cuesta, 2009).

Decisive experiments have made it possible to demonstrate that several diurnal rhythms originate in an animal's own organism. These are known as *endogenous* circadian rhythms. In other words, an animal does not need to be exposed to the environment for these rhythms to exist. This indicates that a true biological clock is at the root of circadian rhythms. In mammals, the basic component of this clock is located in small bilateral structures called the suprachiasmatic nuclei of the hypothalamus. These nuclei control the temporal organization of diurnal rhythms in the entire organism. Each is smaller than one cubic millimetre in size, but is made up of approximately 45,000 neurons. The nuclei are found in the centre of the brain, in the anterior hypothalamus, just above the optic chiasm (Figure 10). Their neurons, among the smallest in the brain, each have a diurnal activity rhythm, indicating that the mechanisms at the origin of circadian rhythms are intracellular. If the suprachiasmatic nuclei of an animal were destroyed, the animal's daily activity and resting rhythm would be disrupted. In such a case, transplanting suprachiasmatic nuclei from a foetus would reset the circadian rhythms, but with the donor's characteristics. Circadian rhythms are therefore genetically determined. The genetic basis of circadian rhythms explains in large part the variability seen in sleep habits among individuals. For example, some people will say they are morning people or evening people, depending on whether they like to go to

THE CENTRAL CLOCK

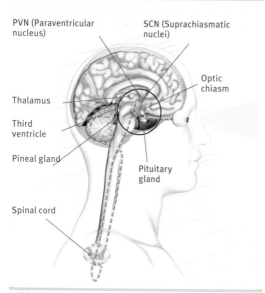

PVN (Paraventricular nucleus)

SCN (Suprachiasmatic nuclei)

Optic chiasm

Thalamus

Third ventricle

Pineal gland

Pituitary gland

Spinal cord

FIGURE 10

bed and get up earlier or later. Figure 11 lets you find out what circadian type (or chronotype) you belong to.

SYNCHRONIZING OUR INNER AND OUTER WORLDS

People placed in a time-isolation environment continue to sleep and wake up every day. This cyclical behaviour is caused by the organism's biological clock. This clock runs according to its own daily rhythm. In fact, the human biological day is very similar to the terrestrial day — on average roughly twenty-four hours and four minutes long. The length of biological days varies from one individual to another and is approximately twenty-three and a half to twenty-four and a half hours long (Gronfier et al., 2007). Since our biological days are slightly different from terrestrial days, we constantly have to reset our

biological clocks to Earth time. To successfully synchronize the length of its biological days with that of terrestrial days, the organism has to decode the signals that tell it about the environmental cycle. In other words, every day, environmental synchronizers called *zeitgebers* (from the German *Zeitgeber*, "giver of time") indicate to individuals' biological clocks the length of the terrestrial day. In all animal species studied to date, the most powerful circadian synchronizer by far is the light-dark cycle.

Our circadian clock nonetheless has natural limits to its ability to adapt to environmental cycles. Thus, if Earth were threatened with destruction and we were offered deportation to another planet, we could get used to a limited number of planetary days. In this scenario, we would have to try to avoid planets with days shorter than twenty-three hours or longer than twenty-seven, since these exceed the circadian clock's entrainment capacity, barring the use of very bright light exposure therapy — and even that might not do the trick.

BODY TEMPERATURE

Core body temperature varies during the day. It reaches its maximum one or two hours before the usual bedtime, and then drops gradually overnight, reaching its minimum one or two hours before we usually get up. The process of falling asleep is accompanied by a loss of heat in the extremities (fingers and toes); this in turn triggers a decrease in core body temperature and promotes sleep.

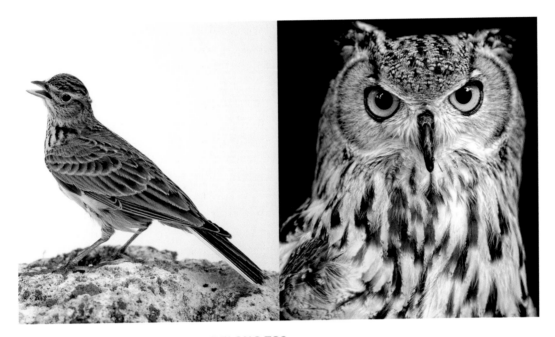

WHICH CHRONOTYPE DO YOU BELONG TO?

Several biological and psychological factors influence our sleep and activity schedule. Thus, some people are early birds while others are night owls. The following questions give an overview of the various chronotypes. Answer as if you are entirely free to plan your day.

	Definitely morning type	Moderately morning type	Neither type	Moderately evening type	Definitely evening type
At what time do you get up naturally?	05:00–06:30	06:30–07:45	07:45–09:45	09:45–11:00	11:00–12:00
At what time do you go to bed naturally?	20:00–21:00	21:00–22:15	22:15–00:30	00:30–01:45	01:45–03:00
At what time do you start to feel tired in the evening?	20:00–21:00	21:00–22:15	22:15–00:45	00:45–02:00	02:00–03:00
At what time of day do you feel you perform best?	5:00–8:00	8:00–10:00	10:00–17:00	17:00–22:00	22:00–05:00

FIGURE 11

Adapted from J. A. Horne and O. Östberg (1976). The full validated test is much longer and is available in the original article.

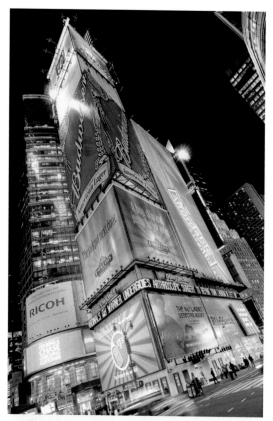

The Circadian Rhythms

Diurnal rhythms are called circadian because they operate on a more or less twenty-four-hour schedule. The Latin roots of this term are circa ("around") and diem ("day"). Figure 12 shows a number of circadian rhythms for a person who has a regular daytime schedule and sleeps at night (Figure 12).

MELATONIN

Melatonin is a hormone secreted by the pineal gland during the night in both diurnal and nocturnal animal species. Its relationship with the sleep-wake cycle and its presumed role in promoting sleep thus depend on the animal. In humans, the secretion of melatonin begins in the evening, a few hours before the usual bedtime. The levels of melatonin in the blood are at their peak in the middle of the night. Then they begin to drop and return to levels that are hard to detect in late morning. They remain very low until the evening.

CORTISOL

Cortisol is a hormone secreted by the adrenal glands. It plays a role in an organism's response to stress. Its secretion varies in the course of a day according to a well-established circadian rhythm. Its blood level is at its peak in the morning at the normal wake time. It drops gradually during the day and reaches its lowest point early in the night, during the first hours of sleep.

The various circadian rhythms work together in the organism to maintain a precise time relationship among themselves and in relation to the sleep/darkness and activity/light rhythm. All of these rhythms are synchronized with the environmental cycle of roughly twenty-four hours, at least if we live on planet Earth! They each have their own variation range and specific maximum and minimum points.

This well-oiled time mechanism ensures the maintenance of good physical and mental health. As a result, even a tiny change or waning over time of one rhythm in relation to another can influence the likelihood of contracting various diseases. The central biological clock is a little like an orchestra conductor directing the rhythm of the organs' functioning, so that they can maintain the right tempo and melody, with the upbeats and downbeats in the right places.

BODY TEMPERATURE AND PLASMA MELATONIN

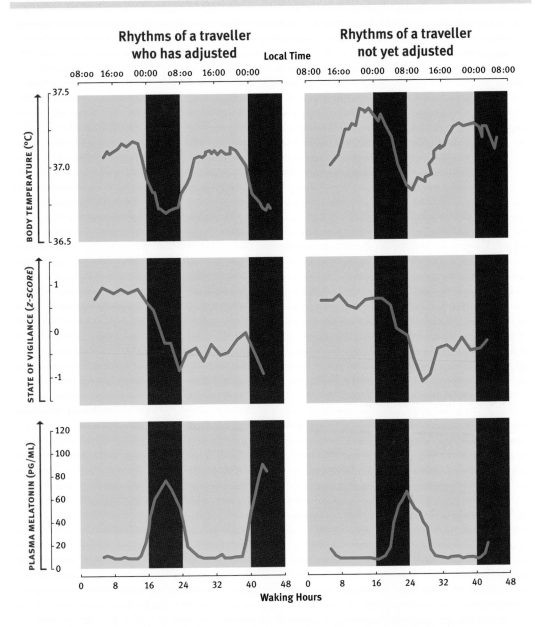

When the adaptation to jet lag is complete, the circadian rhythms reset themselves appropriately in relation to the sleep episode. This is the case of the traveller on the left, who has adjusted well to the Montreal-London time difference. The traveller on the right has not adjusted and his rhythms occur too late in relation to his sleep episode in London.

FIGURE 12   Adapted from Dr. D.B. Boivin, 2002

SHEDDING LIGHT ON OUR BODY CLOCK

Because of their anatomical location, the suprachiasmatic nuclei receive visual information from both retinas. This information about light levels is transmitted from the retina to the suprachiasmatic nuclei along a direct and very powerful neuronal pathway, called the retinohypothalamic tract. The neuronal mechanisms involved in synchronizing the body clock by means of light are different from the mechanisms involved in vision, to the point where it's even possible for someone who is blind to be sensitive to light as a circadian synchronizer (Czeisler et al., 1995). You can therefore be blind neurologically, but be sighted in circadian terms.

The retina's cones and rods transfer to the brain the visual information that enables us to see. These photoreceptors, however, also play a secondary role in entraining the biological clock to light. In fact, a group of specialized ganglion cells have been discovered that are sensitive to light. They send images to the suprachiasmatic nuclei, which makes it possible to adjust their rhythms to the light/dark cycle. These cells contain a photopigment, melanopsin, which is sensitive to short wavelengths, or blue light. The ganglion cells with melanopsin are the principal gateway through which light influences circadian rhythms. That said, the absence of these cells (as in some transgenic mice) does not eliminate the possibility of using light to entrain the body clock. We know that information from the cones and rods can also act on the circadian pacemaker. The fact that photic information reaches the biological clock through two channels guarantees additional security in case one component fails.

Light has a biological effect on the circadian rhythms. For example, when individuals expose themselves to bright light at night, the pineal gland's melatonin secretion is inhibited (Figure 13). The brighter the light, the more pronounced the reduction in melatonin will be. This is why we recommend to insomniac patients who get up during the night to keep the lights as low as possible.

Light has another biological effect on the circadian system. It enables us to adjust its schedule, and in a way to cross internal time zones. The effect of light varies depending on when we are exposed to it, a relationship described by a phase response curve. Thus, being exposed to bright light late in the evening and early in the night displaces the circadian oscillation to a later time. This is called a phase delay and is similar to the adaptation to jet lag following an airplane flight westward. In contrast, being exposed to bright light at the end of the night and early in the morning shifts the circadian oscillation to an earlier time. This is then called a circadian phase advance and is similar to the adaptation to jet lag after an airplane flight eastward (Figure 14). A dose-response curve showing this effect on human beings has been described and indicates that the circadian system is very sensitive to the biological effect of light, even the artificial light produced by ordinary house lamps.

THE OTHER BODY CLOCK SYNCHRONIZERS

Other synchronizers, called non-photic because light is not involved, have been identified. Among these are exercise, social interactions, and meal times. These

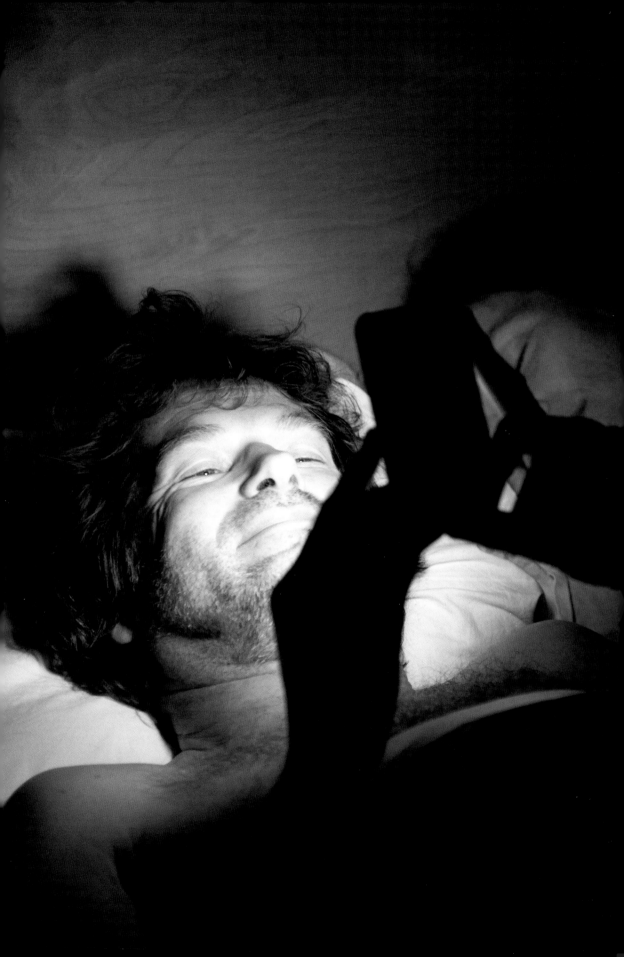

LIGHT AND THE BODY CLOCK

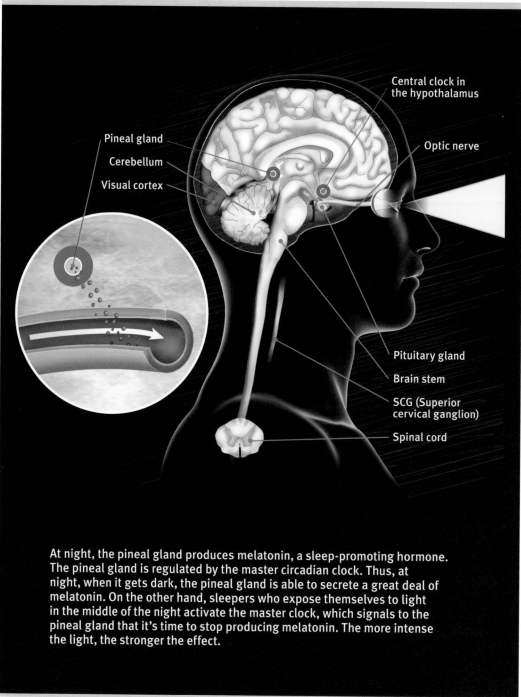

At night, the pineal gland produces melatonin, a sleep-promoting hormone. The pineal gland is regulated by the master circadian clock. Thus, at night, when it gets dark, the pineal gland is able to secrete a great deal of melatonin. On the other hand, sleepers who expose themselves to light in the middle of the night activate the master clock, which signals to the pineal gland that it's time to stop producing melatonin. The more intense the light, the stronger the effect.

FIGURE 13

might explain why some blind people, insensitive to the entrainment effect of light on their body clock, manage to maintain a twenty-four hour rhythm and adapt to their environment. Overall, these non-photic synchronizers are weaker and their effects less clear than those of light. To date, the most studied non-photic synchronizer is melatonin.

Melatonin can entrain the circadian clock and shift its oscillation to other internal time zones. A phase response curve has been described to illustrate the circadian entrainment effect of melatonin. This curve is almost the mirror image of the phase response curve to light. Taking melatonin pills late in the afternoon and in the evening can shift the biological rhythms to an earlier time of day, somewhat like a plane trip eastward. This is called a circadian phase advance. In contrast, taking melatonin pills in the morning and the early afternoon can shift the circadian rhythms to a later time of day, somewhat like a plane trip westward. This is called a circadian phase delay.

PHASE RESPONSE CURVE SHOWING THE ENTERTAINMENT EFFECT OF LIGHT ON THE BIOLOGICAL CLOCK

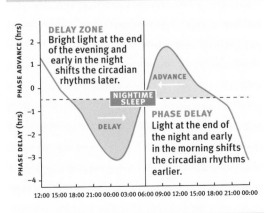

FIGURE 14   Adapted from Khalsa et al., 2003.

THE VARIOUS HUMAN CIRCADIAN CLOCKS

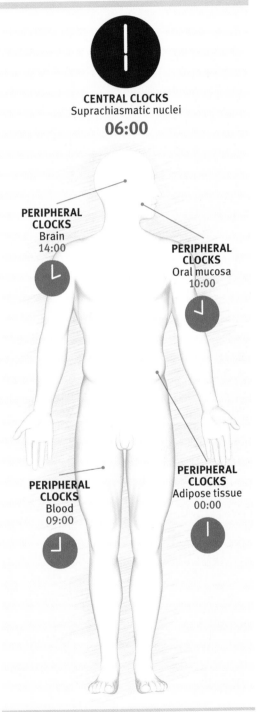

CENTRAL CLOCKS
Suprachiasmatic nuclei
06:00

PERIPHERAL CLOCKS
Brain
14:00

PERIPHERAL CLOCKS
Oral mucosa
10:00

PERIPHERAL CLOCKS
Blood
09:00

PERIPHERAL CLOCKS
Adipose tissue
00:00

FIGURE 15

That said, the "phase delay" section of the melatonin phase response curve is less well defined than its "phase advance" section.

THE TWO PROCESSES REGULATING THE SLEEP-WAKE CYCLE

The quality and duration of sleep rely on a balance between two processes. One of these processes, called the homeostatic process, responds to fatigue accumulated during the day. Thus, we sleep in order to recover from the day's fatigue, which is proportional to the length of the waking period, that is, the time that has elapsed since we woke up. Sleep pressure will be even greater if there was already a sleep debt. This process is also called the S process, for sleep.

The other process is called Circadian — or process C — and is influenced by the sleep schedule. The biological clock sends very strong sleep signals at the end of the night, about one or two hours before our normal wake-up time. Conversely, it sends very strong wake-up signals at the end of the day, approximately one or two hours before our normal bedtime. This circadian-influenced schedule, at first surprising, is in fact the perfect complement to the homeostatic sleep process.

We go to sleep at night because we have accumulated significant fatigue during the day — this is the S process. We get rid of most of this fatigue in the first half of the night, but we still sleep roughly eight hours thanks to our biological clock sending strong sleep signals at the end of the night — this is the C process. We get up in the morning rested and we can function throughout the morning because we have slept well the night before (S process). At the end of the day, we have again accumulated quite a lot of fatigue, but we manage to stay awake, as our biological clock takes over and sends stronger and stronger wake-up signals (C process). During the day, the S and C processes take turns, so that we can stay awake for sixteen hours straight. They do the same at night, which means we can sleep eight consecutive hours, when everything is going well.

Some people feel a drop in energy after the noon meal. This is because at that point several hours of fatigue have already accumulated while the biological clock is not quite awake, and the digestive process can make this desire to fall asleep, known as the post-lunch dip, hard to resist (Chapter 5).

CIRCADIAN RHYTHM DISORDERS

Well-orchestrated "circadian music" goes along with good physical and mental health. When a circadian rhythm kicks in at the wrong time, "wrong notes" can be heard. The normally well-oiled biological clock mechanism becomes less efficient. This happens when people's natural biological rhythms are disrupted by a particular way of life or for psychological reasons.

Circadian rhythm disorders are either called extrinsic, since they are caused by disruptions outside the circadian system itself, or intrinsic, stemming from an internal biological disruption of the circadian rhythms. For example, difficulties in adjusting to night work and jet lag are extrinsic circadian rhythm disorders. Intrinsic disorders, on the other hand, include extreme sleep schedule and irregular sleep-wake schedule disruptions. There is no doubt

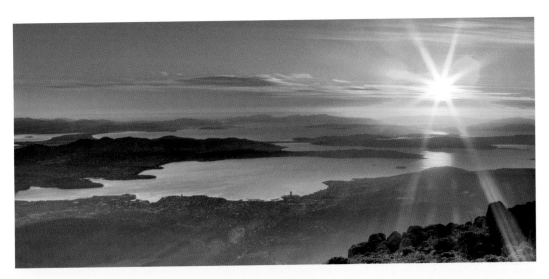

The Genetic Basis of Circadian Rhythms

The study of several animal species, including humans, has made it possible to identify a series of genes called circadian clock genes. These are required to generate and maintain circadian rhythms in a stable environment (for example in constant darkness without alternating days and nights). These genes and the proteins they encode are an integral part of the positive and negative feedback loops at the heart of circadian rhythms (Cermakian and Boivin, 2003). In mammals, the circadian clock genes were first noted in the suprachiasmatic nuclei of the hypothalamus. But these rhythms have since been detected in several organs in the body, such as the liver, heart and kidneys, as well as in the blood cells and other regions of the brain.

Scientists believe that our circadian system is made up of a central clock, located in the suprachiasmatic nuclei of the hypothalamus, and peripheral clocks in other regions of the brain and body (Figure 15). In addition, these clocks continue to oscillate even when they are studied in culture outside the organism (Brown et al., 2008). In the body, the central clock may synchronize the peripheral clocks. The mechanisms underlying these phenomena are currently being studied. Various synchronizers can have different effects on the central clock and the peripheral clocks. It's possible, for example, to regulate the peripheral clocks independently of the central clock by limiting access to food. Other genes (roughly 5 to 10 percent of the whole genome) vary in the course of a day. The genes controlled by the circadian clock genes are expressed differently in each organ. Intensive research is trying to clarify the roles of these rhythms in how each tissue functions and their influence on the onset of various diseases. In short, it is these circadian genes and other genes regulating the homeostasis of sleep that determine our sleep behaviour.

Melatonin

Melatonin is a hormone secreted by the pineal gland at night. Its effect is seen in the entire organism through its action on melatonin receptors. These are found in most organs, glands, and tissues, in the retina and throughout the central nervous system, including the suprachiasmatic nuclei. Melatonin secretion has a circadian rhythm that depends on the master biological clock, since a series of indirect neuronal connections running through the spinal cord links the biological clock to the pineal gland (Figure 13). The secretion of melatonin tells the organism when night begins and ends.

Although melatonin is a hormone, it's freely available in pill form in the natural products sections of many drugstores. Despite this very easy access, the long-term effects on health, the dosing schedule, and the optimal doses of melatonin have not been systematically studied. The doses tested in scientific studies range from 0.3 to 10 mg and are taken over several days.

Melatonin has two main effects on human rhythms. First, it helps in falling asleep and staying asleep. This is its hypnotic or sedative effect, which is accompanied by a decrease in core body temperature. Taking melatonin pills in the middle of the afternoon (a time when levels are undetectable) will cause drowsiness and help put you to sleep at that time. Taking melatonin at bedtime (when we are already producing it) will have a less noticeable effect in a healthy person. Various pharmaceutical products like ramelteon (whose sale in Canada is currently prohibited) act on melatonin receptors and have been developed for patients suffering from sleep and circadian rhythm disorders.

Secondly, melatonin in pill form can shift the timing of circadian rhythms, with this effect depending on when the medication is taken. This is called the chronobiotic effect.

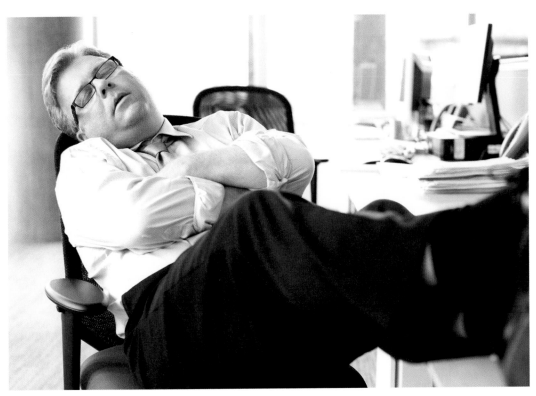

that the technological progress that led to the invention of electricity and the electric light bulb, as well as modern life, play a major role in disrupting the sleep habits of modern human beings. A very long time ago, "midnight" meant the middle of the night. Now, many of us are not even in bed by that time, while others are on their way to work!

NIGHT WORK AND SHIFT WORK

When people stay awake all night and sleep during the day, they force their organism to remain active at a time when it's programmed to sleep, and to sleep at a time when it's programmed to be awake. The daytime sleep of night workers is often shorter and more disrupted than that of daytime workers. A study by Statistics Canada shows that 34 percent of shift workers say they have had problems getting to sleep and staying asleep, compared with 26 percent of workers with a regular daytime schedule (Hurst, 2008). Night workers often get to sleep easily in the morning, because they have built up significant fatigue the previous day and during their work overnight. However, they often wake up too soon, since their biological clock sends wake-up signals to their brain, signals that become progressively stronger late in the morning and in the afternoon. Night workers thus accumulate a daily sleep debt of between one and three hours. In addition to losing several hours of sleep time, the structure of their daytime sleep is disrupted, compared with nighttime sleep. It's not uncommon for night workers to get their sleep in several stretches between shifts.

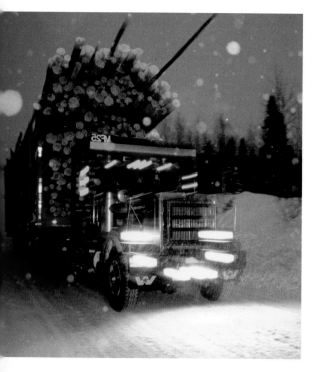

seven times as many medical errors due to fatigue as their more rested counterparts (Barger, 2006).

Turning night into day disrupts the harmony among the various circadian rhythms. This means that night workers will be awake at the same time they are secreting melatonin, making them less vigilant. And they will try to sleep during the day while secreting cortisol, a stress hormone, instead of melatonin. It is of course better to sleep while secreting more melatonin and be awake while secreting more cortisol (as is the case for day workers). Over time, the circadian rhythms can partially adapt to a daily rhythm that's out of sync. But in less than one night worker in twenty are circadian rhythms fully adapted to night work.

At night, workers try to be productive, while their biological clock is sending powerful sleep signals. These signals, combined with significant fatigue from an accumulated lack of sleep and an extended period of wakefulness, have an impact on levels of vigilance and impair their physical and mental acuity. They are therefore more likely to make mistakes and have accidents, especially at the end of the night. These risks increase as shifts get longer and there is less time to rest (Boivin et al., 2010). The most recent Canadian data (2006) indicate that fatigue at the wheel is a factor in almost 22 percent of fatal accidents and in 20 percent of all accidents resulting in bodily harm. Studies carried out on locomotive engineers show that they experience severe drowsiness more than half the time when they work at night. Resident doctors exhausted by an overloaded work schedule appear to make

JET LAG

Travellers who take flights from east to west cross time zones quickly. They force their bodies to adjust to a different local time. During a trip eastward (such as a Montreal–London flight), the body has to learn to go to bed and get up five hours earlier in London than in Montreal (Figure 12). Gradually, the central biological clock will align the body's rhythms with the new location. This adaptation process actually takes place in the country of arrival. However, this adjustment is not instantaneous and we have to expect on average one day of adaptation per time zone crossed before we are completely resynchronized.

The opposite adaptation occurs during the return trip to the point of departure. The biological clock then has to delay diurnal rhythms so that they oscillate five hours later in Montreal than they did in London. Throughout the adaptation period, both going and coming, travellers experience a transitory period when both sleeping and waking are disrupted. This is called jet lag disorder (Arendt, 2009). Tolerance to jet lag and its accompanying lack of sleep vary enormously from person to person, but the degree of disruption experienced depends on the number of time zones crossed. Trips eastward require a more difficult adaptation than trips westward, but further research is needed to better understand why this is so.

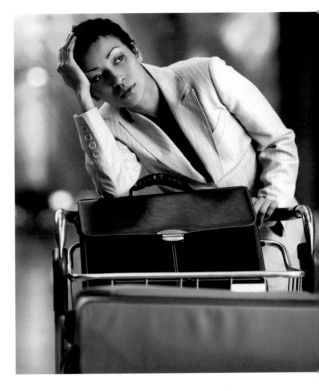

SLEEP SCHEDULE DISORDERS

Sleep schedules or habits vary a great deal from one individual to another (Figure 11). "Morning" people like to go to bed and get up early. They are more productive and creative in the morning and therefore more tired in the evening. "Night" people prefer to go to bed and get up late. They are slower off the mark in the morning and become more energetic in the afternoon and evening. They are also wide awake in the evening and go to bed late. There are all sorts of variations between these two types of sleep schedule. When sleep habits are more extreme and inflexible, they cause social adaptation problems. This is called sleep schedule disorder. Patients who are extreme "night people" suffer from what is called delayed sleep phase disorder. They take several hours to get to sleep and find it very hard to get out of bed in the morning. Their body has trouble getting to sleep before 3:00 to 6:00 a.m. and waking up earlier than between 10:00 in the morning and 3:00 in the afternoon. This type of disorder often results in a very irregular sleep schedule; this means that sleep is in very short supply on work days and is made up for on days off. This gap between a socially imposed sleep schedule and our biological schedule is called social jet lag (Wittmann et al., 2006). It's a condition that can seriously disrupt people's quality of life and is widely observed in extreme "night owls."

A natural period of delayed sleep phase disorder occurs in adolescence. Adolescents' biological clocks are naturally set to another time zone, much farther west than that of their parents. During the week, adolescents therefore suffer from serious sleep deprivation, since they have to cut their nights short to get to class. They often make up this accumulated fatigue by sleeping later on weekends. The result is family tension triggered by teenagers staying in bed too late. Fortunately, sleep schedules become regular in early adulthood for most people. Some patients, however, retain this skewed sleep pattern even as adults, causing them problems at work unless they work in the evening or at night. It's estimated that approximately 7.3 percent of teenagers, compared with 0.13 to 3.1 percent of the adult population, have delayed sleep phase disorder.

Advanced sleep phase disorder is the opposite problem — an abnormally early sleep schedule. Patients with this disorder have trouble staying awake later than 6:00 to 9:00 p.m. and they get up unusually early, between 2:00 and 5:00 a.m. This disorder affects about 1 percent of middle-aged adults and the likelihood of developing it increases with age. It's generally seen in older patients, although cases of a number of families in which several members have advanced sleep phase disorder have been reported. In these cases, this is a hereditary disorder affecting the circadian clock genes.

Some patients have another unusual and very serious sleep schedule disorder known as non-twenty-four-hour sleep-wake disorder. These patients have a biological clock that cannot seem to adapt to the external environment and "freely runs on its own schedule," based on its internal biological days. These patients are constantly out of alignment with their environment and are unable to adapt to it. This disorder may affect nearly 50 percent of blind patients, when they are insensitive to light as a circadian synchronizer. Sighted patients can also be affected, but much more rarely.

There is one more circadian rhythm disorder, called irregular sleep-wake disorder. This disorder is most commonly seen in geriatric populations living in institutions. Patients sleep in three or more short episodes, spread over the day and night. A fundamental problem with the workings of the biological clock is suspected. For example, a loss of nearly 40 percent of neurons has been observed in the suprachiasmatic nuclei of patients who have died of Alzheimer's disease. Analysis of these patients' brains has enabled us to detect a disruption between their central and peripheral brain clocks (Chapter 3).

Circadian rhythm disorders are typically hard to treat. A rigorous review of sleep hygiene and daily schedules is therefore important (Chapter 4). The doctor may suggest a therapeutic approach combining chronotherapy — based on the gradual modification of sleep schedules, diet, and social interactions — light therapy — using a bright light lamp — and the use of products like melatonin or sleeping pills.

What Should You Take Away From This Chapter?

- Circadian rhythms are biological and psychological rhythms of about twenty-four hours and include hormone secretion, the tendency to sleep, and body temperature.

- The secretion of the hormones melatonin and cortisol follows a well-established circadian rhythm. Melatonin levels are at their peak in the middle of the night, whereas cortisol levels reach theirs when we get up in the morning.

- A real biological clock controls our body's circadian rhythms. Located in the centre of the brain, it's connected to the retina by a very powerful neuronal pathway, called the retinohypothalamic tract.

- Our body has a central clock and peripheral clocks located elsewhere in the brain and body.

- Our internal biological days are slightly shorter or longer than twenty-four hours. Every day, we adjust our internal biological rhythms to terrestrial days. To do this, our biological clock decodes signals from the external world that tell it the time of day and the length of terrestrial days.

- Difficulty in maintaining a socially acceptable sleep schedule is a sign of a circadian rhythm disorder. The cause of these disorders may lie outside the body, in the case of those triggered by night work or jet lag, or stem from an intrinsic biological tendency to live according to a different schedule. Examples of this include advanced or delayed sleep phase disorder, non-twenty-four-hour sleep-wake disorder, and irregular sleep-wake disorder.

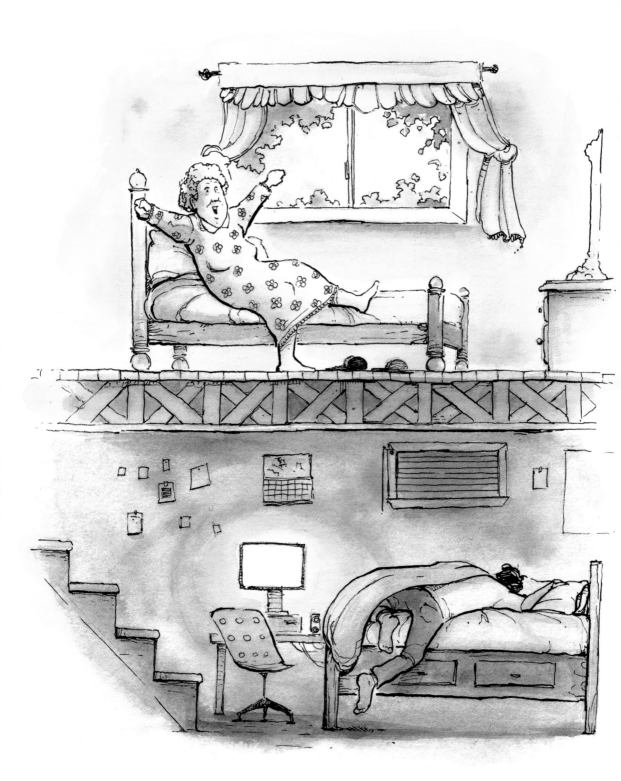

A morning for everyone.

CHAPTER 3

Searching for the Fountain of Youth

Sleep at All Ages

Our sleep undergoes significant changes in our lifetime, both in its internal organization and in its schedule over the course of a day. Considerable variation exists among individuals and is also obvious when we look at sleep and aging. The decline in slow wave sleep with age is more noticeable in patients with sleep disorders or debilitating illnesses like Alzheimer's disease. In addition, men's and women's sleep patterns change in different ways. This chapter explains how sleep changes over a lifetime. This information is important in distinguishing conditions that reflect normal changes from those requiring medical attention.

INFANTS

As young parents know, the sleep of newborn babies is very different from that of children and adults. At birth, sleep is not yet fully organized into a twenty-four-hour sleep-wake cycle and does not have the typical stages of sleep found in adults. Instead, it's divided into calm and active sleep phases, interrupted by periods of wakefulness during which all attention is focussed on feeding. This is the breast-feeding or bottle-feeding phase. Since the human brain is complex, it takes time to reach maturity, and sleep will continue to change throughout this maturation process. Human beings, a so-called altricial animal species (whose maturation is incomplete at birth), will spend a great deal more time in REM sleep (or in active sleep, in the case of infants) than precocial species, whose brain is mature at birth. The proportion of time infants spend in REM sleep is therefore substantial, but decreases gradually as the brain develops. Interestingly, newborns go from a waking state to REM sleep without transition, a condition deemed pathological in adults.

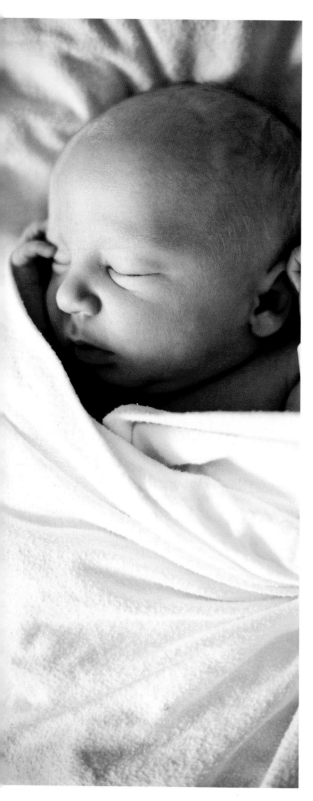

Between two and six months, the phases of calm sleep begin to develop into the other stages of sleep. Slow wave sleep appears when the brain has developed sufficiently to generate slow delta waves. Exactly how circadian rhythms develop has not been studied very much in newborns, but it looks like the rhythm of melatonin and cortisol secretion begins to become apparent at around three months of age. Through breast-feeding, the newborn is exposed to the natural secretion rhythm of its mother's melatonin, since this hormone is found in breast milk. It's still not known whether children who are breastfed develop their circadian rhythms faster than those who are bottle-fed. Given our current state of knowledge, taking melatonin pills must not even be considered if you are breast-feeding, and they certainly must not be given to newborns. In fact, very little data is available on whether or not melatonin pills are harmful to infants. Furthermore, mothers who take melatonin pills may reduce their levels of prolactin, a hormone important for producing breast milk. Women planning to get pregnant should also avoid taking melatonin pills, as this may increase the risk of child development disorders.

Many questions about how sleep and circadian rhythms develop in newborns are still unanswered. We recommend that parents begin exposing their babies as soon as possible to a regular cycle of light and darkness. Doing so will quickly establish good habits in terms of exposing the biological clock to environmental synchronizers.

CHILDREN

During childhood, sleep undergoes major changes. Typically, children's sleep involves a great amount of slow wave sleep. In fact, it's during childhood that human beings get the most slow wave sleep; the proportion of this stage of sleep compared to other stages of sleep decreases gradually with age (Kurt et al., 2010). As we saw in Chapter 1, slow wave sleep and the slow waves that characterize it are associated with sleep's recovery function. During slow wave sleep, there is considerable secretion of growth hormone, which promotes growth and tissue repair. Sleep disruptions in children are thus of concern to scientists because of the possible harmful effects on growth and intellectual development. Good sleep habits, with regular bedtimes and wake times, and, above all, enough sleep time, are important.

It should also be noted that it's during slow wave sleep that phenomena such as episodes of sleepwalking and night terrors occur (Chapter 9). These are in fact very common in children and are part of brain maturation, given that a very large amount of slow wave sleep is typical in this phase of life.

The arousal threshold for a child in slow wave sleep is quite high and they often appear confused when awakened. This confusion is called sleep inertia. This is why it takes a while for children to become fully awake when they have been sleeping deeply. Incidentally, it's not dangerous to wake up a sleepwalking child and we should not hesitate to do so if the child is in a dangerous situation, about to jump out of a window, for example. Fortunately, these situations rarely occur with children. It's also possible to try to suggest to children who are still half asleep that they should go back to their own bed and to reassure them that there are no monsters under the bed or in the closet. Night fears can sometimes become a strategy for getting into bed with parents, but it's important for children to learn to sleep by themselves. A solid balance between reassurance and firmness will help manage these episodes.

It's also important for children and their parents to establish a regular bedtime and wake-up routine. Children who go to bed after 9:00 p.m. or at irregular times are roughly twice as likely to be short of sleep as children who go to bed earlier or at regular times (Owens et al., 2011).

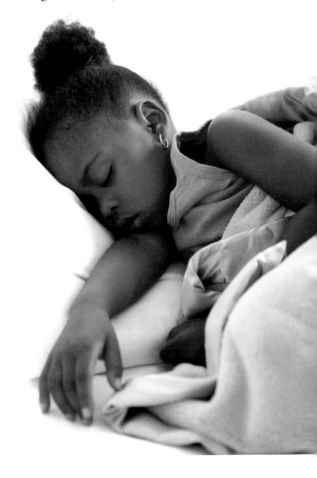

ADOLESCENTS

During puberty, adolescents go through a period of intense hormonal changes they have to learn to cope with. Their bodies change during this period and they are absorbed by personal concerns and a desire to be independent from their parents. Their sexual urges become stronger and their interests and social interactions change. This period often involves tensions with family members and peers. Their sleep habits also change considerably; this new sleep schedule is in fact a delayed sleep phase disorder, as we saw in Chapter 2. This is a normal period of change in the sleep schedule that is usually temporary and related to puberty. During this period there is a natural tendency to go to bed and get up at times that are later and out of sync with social norms.

Adolescents' sleep thus appears to be more in line with that of adults living in time zones further west. For example, a teenager living in Montreal or Quebec City might go to sleep naturally at the same time as an adult living in Vancouver or California. The reasons behind these changes require more scientific study. They may stem from a temporary increase in the length of internal biological days, exposure to light later in the evening, altered sensitivity to the effect of light on the biological clock or heightened resistance to lack of sleep (Hagenauer et al., 2009). Nonetheless, teenagers continue to live in a society that requires them to get up at times that are earlier than those determined by their biological clocks. Typically, teenagers accumulate a significant sleep debt during weekdays because of school obligations, a situation that can greatly affect their attention span in class, how well they retain knowledge in the long term and their results at school. On weekends, teenagers tend to sleep much later in the morning to make up the sleep lost during the week. Bedtimes and wake-up times are frequently several hours later on Saturdays and Sundays because there are no social obligations. On those days, teenagers may pursue activities that make their tendency to sleep later even worse, for example, playing video or computer games for much of the night.

This often aggravates family tensions, with teenagers perceived as being lazy, disorganized slobs who lie around in bed all day long. A discussion between parents and teenagers of the biological reasons for delayed sleep phase disorder may be beneficial for all family members. In addition, major differences in sleep schedules between the week and weekend should be avoided as much as possible. The later that bedtimes and wake times are on the weekend, the later teenagers are exposed to light. This delayed light exposure schedule resets the biological clock even later (like a plane trip westward). As a result, it's that much more difficult for teenagers to readjust to a socially acceptable sleep schedule on Sunday night.

It is possible to modify our light exposure schedule so that our biological clock is better attuned to our environment. This approach consists of increasing exposure to bright light in the morning and reducing light levels in the evening. In theory, light therapy lamps could even be considered; this approach is actually being studied. For the time being, this treatment is usually recommended for treating

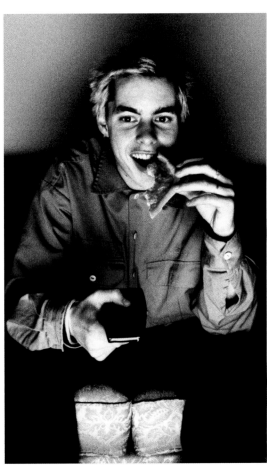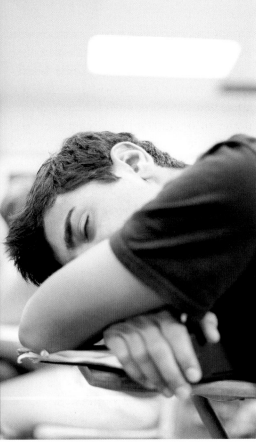

SLEEP 101 FOR TEENAGERS

1. Follow the advice in "The insomniac's ten commandments" (Chapter 4).

2. Keep light levels as low as possible during the evening.

3. Expose yourself to sunlight early in the day, especially in late morning and early afternoon.

4. Schedule your physical exercise early in the day. Avoid intensive practice and sports games late in the evening.

5. Avoid playing on the Internet late in the evening.

6. Turn off cell phones and SMS at night.

7. Try to relax if you wake up at night. Avoid stimulating activities like watching action movies and using the Internet.

8. Decorate your bedroom to make it a relaxing and restful place. Do your homework and watch movies in another room.

9. Avoid drinking too many energy drinks during the day.

10. Keep your sleep schedule as regular as possible on weekends and weekdays.

FIGURE 16

persistent circadian rhythm disorders. A thorough review of sleep hygiene would be a good idea at this age, to keep the condition from getting worse (Figure 16). A morning walk after waking up would also be helpful, but good luck getting your teenager on board!

YOUNG ADULTS

The fog of adolescence lifts and adulthood finally begins to take shape, along with free access to all kinds of bars. Ah! The twenties! These days, few young adults start families in this phase of their lives. Most of them are still studying or working at paid jobs. In general, young adults sleep well and their out-of-sync sleep schedule gets back on track. Bedtimes and wake times tend to become regular and are greatly influenced by young adults' social activities. Nonetheless, many young adults are socially active and go to bed later on weekends. As a result, some of them (especially those without many social obligations) continue to have a delayed sleep schedule, just like in adolescence. This adult population is at greatest risk of delayed sleep phase disorder, causing those affected to have trouble falling asleep and getting up in the morning.

MEN COMPARED TO WOMEN

In adulthood, there are a number of differences between men's and women's sleep. Women of all ages tend to sleep a little more than men. However, they are twice as likely to have insomnia. Hormonal factors seem to partly explain this. Hormonal and body temperature fluctuations occur during the menstrual cycle (Figure 17). In addition, estrogen, progesterone, and testosterone receptors are located on the neurons of the suprachiasmatic nuclei of the hypothalamus, the central biological clock. It has also been observed that the structure of brain waves during sleep varies in the course of the menstrual cycle. For example, during the luteal phase there are more rapid beta-type waves, indicating a lighter state of sleep.

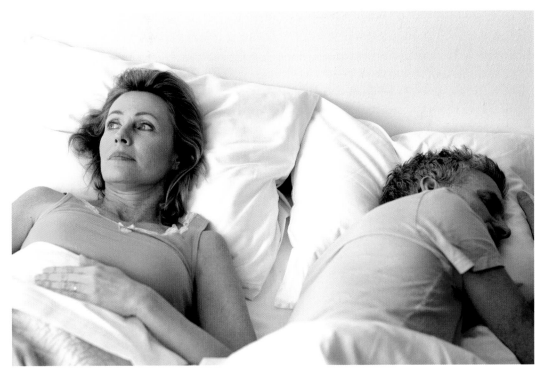

More sleep spindles, resulting from activation loops between the deep areas of the brain (thalamus) and the superficial areas (the cerebral cortex), are also seen. These spindles might indicate that progesterone plays a protective role during this phase of the menstrual cycle.

There is some evidence to suggest differences in men's and women's circadian rhythms. For example, women tend to go to bed and get up earlier, and thus to be "morning people" more often than men. On average, melatonin secretion occurs earlier during the sleep episode in women than in men (Cain et al., 2010). Recent studies have shown that the length of women's biological days is on average six minutes shorter than men's (Duffy et al., 2011). This difference might explain, in part, the shift of women's circadian rhythms to an earlier time of day. These studies have also shown that about one

woman in three, compared with one man in seven, has biological days shorter than twenty-four hours. More studies will be needed to understand the differences between men and women in terms of how their biological clocks operate and what the repercussions are for their sleep. This is an important point, since there are twice as many women as men with insomnia (Buysse et al., 2008). Furthermore, we know that sleep disorders are a risk factor for the onset of depression (Chapter 6).

During their lifetimes, women undergo major changes related to their reproductive system. At the end of their forties or beginning of their fifties, their reproductive system gradually stops functioning. A period of pre-menopause precedes menopause, during which irregular menstrual cycles occur and are further and further apart. Menopause is officially confirmed when menstrual periods have not occurred for at least twelve months. These changes are accompanied by physical changes that can also disrupt the quality of sleep. Insomnia disorders are in fact reported by 40 to 50 percent of menopausal women, compared with 30 percent in their reproductive years. Despite these hormonal changes, the amount of slow wave sleep seems to remain steady in women longer than it does in men. Studies even show an increase in length of sleep and in slow wave sleep, but a lower degree of satisfaction with sleep during this period (Sowers et al., 2008). Among the factors that disrupt sleep are hot flashes, which aren't exactly a recipe for comfort. They strike repeatedly both night and day and can greatly disturb sleep. It may be useful to talk about this problem with your doctor, who might suggest taking a sleeping pill or hormone replacement therapy — taking hormones to counter the ailments associated with natural age-related hormonal decline. A word to spouses: mood swings and irritability

can occur in this phase of women's lives, and this personality change is likely to be made worse by sleep disruptions.

MATURE ADULTS

People today often start their families later than their grandparents did. The sleep of new parents who have a first child when they are between thirty-five and forty-five has already begun to change. It's more fragile than at twenty-five, even before the newborn arrives, with its nighttime feedings and sleepless nights. In fact, measurable changes occur in the structure of sleep after our thirties (Carrier et al., 2011). Over time, there is less slow wave sleep and its efficiency drops in most people. Sleep schedules change with age, with people tending to fall asleep and get up earlier. The aging of sleep is gradual and ongoing; it begins early in life, and how fast the process unfolds varies by individual. It's faster

TEMPERATURE, HORMONES, AND SLEEP DURING THE MENSTRUAL CYCLE

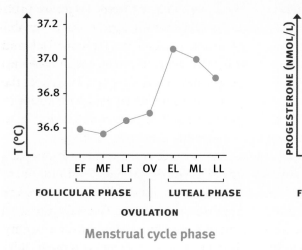
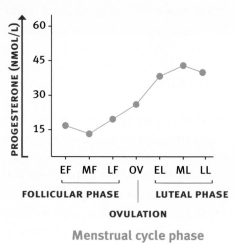

FIGURE 17   Adapted from Schechler et al., 2012.

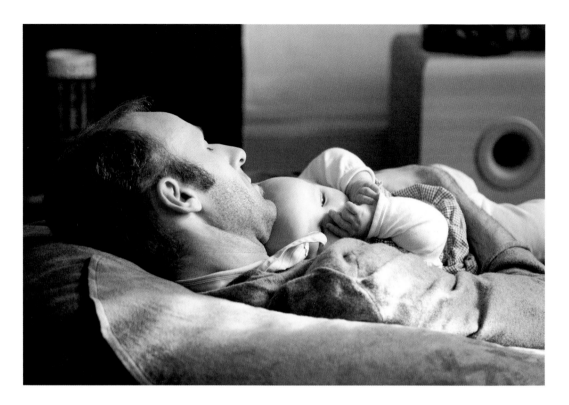

in some people and slower in others. It's difficult to fully identify the factors contributing to individual differences in the sleep aging process, but maintaining good lifestyle habits and eliminating factors that can cause illness, such as smoking, excessive alcohol consumption, drugs, and a sedentary lifestyle, are definitely recommended.

THE ELDERLY

The sleep aging process continues and becomes more pronounced over the course of a lifetime. After age sixty, sleep is lighter and punctuated by frequent awakenings, and features fewer sleep spindles and less slow wave sleep. The decline in slow wave sleep may indicate a disrupted restructuring, during sleep, of synaptic connections among neurons. This is an important

brain recovery process (Chapter 5) and its weakening with age may contribute to the cognitive decline noted as people age. Meanwhile, the proportion of REM sleep remains about the same in healthy older people. It drops dramatically, however, in those with dementia-type cognitive problems. There is thus a great deal of variability in sleep quality among individuals and it is often affected by the health problems people develop as they age. With age, the period during the day when it's easier to get to sleep shifts to an earlier time, and this schedule becomes more rigid.

As they age, many people will complain of fatigue during the day and indulge in daytime naps, especially if they have the opportunity to do so. That said, the total amount of sleep obtained over a twenty-four hour period seems to remain quite steady with age. It's just that the biological

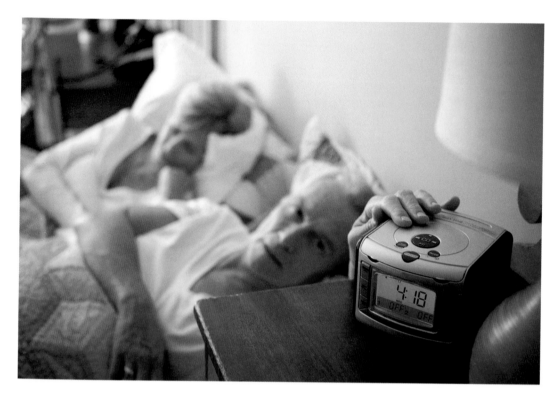

clock resets itself differently with respect to the sleep schedule. Melatonin secretion reaches its peak early in the day, but later in the sleep episode in older people, compared with younger people. This may be related to decreased sensitivity to the effect of light on the biological clock. In comparison, the length of internal biological days is quite stable throughout life. A number of studies have underlined a reduction in the amplitude of several diurnal rhythms with age, including those of body temperature and the secretion of melatonin, cortisol, and growth hormone. At the same time, there is still controversy over whether or not in healthy people circadian rhythms become weaker with age. Cases have in fact been reported of "super old people" with very strong rhythms even at an advanced age! Lastly, with age, there is an increased likelihood of developing

sleep disorders like sleep apnea (Chapter 8) and periodic leg movements during sleep (Chapter 9).

SLEEP AND ALZHEIMER'S DISEASE

Alzheimer's disease is a degenerative brain disease that leads to severe dementia. Approximately one Canadian in twenty over sixty-five and one in four over eighty-five has the disease. Diagnosis is confirmed by autopsy, as the brains of patients who die from this disease contain many amyloid plaques and neurofibrillary tangles that contribute to the death of neurons. This process is particularly evident in the cerebral cortex, especially in the frontal and mediotemporal regions, areas of the brain important for intellectual reasoning, language, learning, and memory.

Gradual dementia is the most devastating aspect of Alzheimer-type senile dementia. Disruptions in the sleep-wake cycle are frequent among people affected; their sleep deteriorates rapidly as the illness progresses and their cognitive functions deteriorate. In most patients with Alzheimer's disease, the diurnal organization of their behaviour is disrupted. Many are agitated at bedtime, a disabling condition called "sundowning syndrome." This condition causes great anxiety and is hard for families to manage. In fact, sleep disorders are one of the most common reasons why patients are institutionalized.

Sleep changes related to aging are more marked in Alzheimer's disease than in healthy older people. In Alzheimer's patients, sleep disruptions are more pronounced than those associated with normal aging of the brain. For example, there is a definite decrease in slow wave sleep and the almost total disappearance of stage 2 sleep, along with a dramatic decrease in its characteristic sleep spindles and K-complexes. Slow wave sleep and stage 2 sleep are replaced by lighter stage 1 sleep. An overall slowdown in brain activity can be seen on an electroencephalogram, both during waking periods and during sleep. This slowdown is especially striking in phases of REM sleep, where dreams occur.

A fragmented sleep-wake cycle is common in Alzheimer's disease and indicates fundamental damage to the circadian system. Anatomically, significant changes are seen in the suprachiasmatic nuclei of the hypothalamus, the master biological clock. The volume of the suprachiasmatic nuclei shrinks in all human beings as they age. In healthy

THE CINGULATE CORTEX

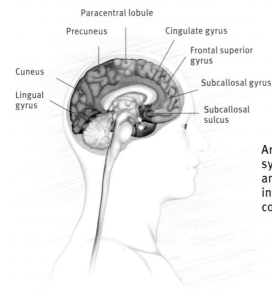

Paracentral lobule
Precuneus
Cingulate gyrus
Frontal superior gyrus
Cuneus
Subcallosal gyrus
Lingual gyrus
Subcallosal sulcus

An important component of the limbic system, which processes emotions, learning and memory, the cingulate cortex is also involved in executive functions (high-level cognitive processes).

FIGURE 18

people it's mainly after the age of eighty that the volume of this structure and the number of neurons it contains appear different from what is seen in people under twenty. In patients with Alzheimer's disease, the suprachiasmatic nuclei are 50 percent smaller than those of people without the disease. This reduction in the size of the nuclei goes along with a decrease in the number of its neurons. The melatonin secretion curve is also dramatically reduced in Alzheimer's disease.

Our research group has recently begun to analyze the brains of patients who died of Alzheimer's disease to compare them with those who died of another cause (Cermakian et al., 2011). This study has shown the presence of circadian clocks in other regions of the brain than the suprachiasmatic nuclei, such as the cingulate cortex (Figure 18) and the nuclei of the bed of the stria terminalis, regions that are important for decision-making and behavioural organization. In Alzheimer's disease, the synchrony amongst these clocks and their relationship with the central clock appears disrupted. These observations confirm that fundamental changes with respect to the circadian rhythms are part of this disease.

Knowing about the natural changes in sleep in the course of a lifetime enables us to better identify those situations that deviate from the norm. This also helps us to maintain realistic expectations with regard to our own sleep. Wanting to sleep like a baby well into old age will generate more anxiety and frustration than benefits. The best attitude to adopt, to sleep as well as possible for as long as possible, is to maintain the best lifestyle habits possible. No matter how hard we try to avoid it, insomnia may occur. That's the subject of the next chapter.

What Should You Take Away From This Chapter?

- Sleep and its schedule undergo major changes with age.

- A delayed sleep phase disorder occurs temporarily during adolescence and may cause family tension.

- Young adults are more likely to have a delayed sleep schedule than are older people, who tend to go to bed and get up earlier.

- At birth and during childhood we see the largest amount of REM sleep and slow wave sleep, respectively.

- Women of all ages sleep slightly more than men. On the other hand, they are more likely to suffer from insomnia. Hormonal factors seem to be involved and appear to affect the circadian and homeostatic sleep processes.

- Healthy older people have better sleep and circadian rhythms than those who develop debilitating diseases.

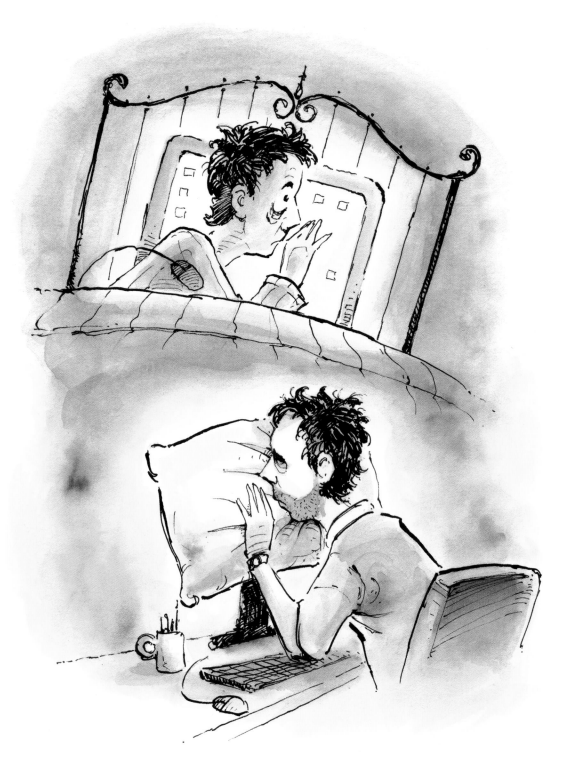

If you have a hard job getting to sleep, you'll wind up sleeping on the job...

CHAPTER 4

When You Miss the Boat

Insomnia and You

Chronic insomnia is by far the most common sleep disorder. It affects patients their whole life long. Approximately 30 to 50 percent of adults are estimated to have symptoms of insomnia at one time or another, and in more than 10 percent of them these problems are believed to be serious and persistent (Budhiraja et al., 2011). The risk of developing insomnia goes up when there are existing medical conditions. The daily lack of sleep that is an integral part of the chronic insomnia profile has major negative impacts on patients' quality of life and increases their risk of developing psychological and physical disorders. Chronic insomnia therefore has serious socioeconomic consequences, since it heightens the risk of developing various health problems, leading to a poorer quality of life and a greater likelihood of absenteeism and traffic accidents (Daley et al., 2009). Fully understanding the factors that influence and disrupt sleep thus enables us to control the risk of disease better. This chapter gives an overview of the causes of insomnia and offers simple advice for sleeping more soundly. We likely won't resolve all problems with this chapter, but the advice it contains might make nighttime easier to deal with for many people.

WHAT IS INSOMNIA?

Insomnia is defined as a recurring difficulty in getting to sleep and staying asleep, despite a suitable sleeping environment. Patients are considered to be suffering from insomnia if they have recurring sleep debt affecting their functioning during the day. For the population in general, it's estimated that an episode of seven to nine hours of sleep each night is optimal in length. This is an average, however, as sleep requirements vary from one person to another. Some people get fewer than six hours' sleep a night without suffering any particular consequences from a lack of sleep. These people are considered to be natural short sleepers. In contrast, other individuals need at least nine hours per night to feel completely rested. As a result, eight hours of nighttime sleep do not totally meet their needs, whereas it would give a natural short sleeper "sleep indigestion." It must be stressed that insomnia is not a diagnosis per se, but rather a medical complaint. When a patient has insomnia, we have to look for the causes in order to fix the problem at its source.

WHAT CAUSES INSOMNIA?

Several sleep disorders, physical illnesses, psychological and psychiatric disorders, and lifestyles can lead to insomnia (Figure 19). These should be identified so as to treat the cause of the problem. In the vast majority of cases, insomnia occurs following a difficult period in a person's life and then persists on its own. During the difficult period (such as following the death of a loved one), the person has trouble sleeping and feels exhausted during the daytime. This lack of sleep and fatigue then become problems in their own right and these people become preoccupied with their lack of sleep and sleepless nights, making them feel worse. Once the difficult period has passed, the sleepless nights may continue for no apparent reason. People then become increasingly preoccupied with their insomnia and the harmful repercussions for their physical and mental health

of a chronic lack of sleep. This creates a vicious circle and insomnia settles in. When the known causes underlying the insomnia no longer exist, it's called chronic psychophysiological insomnia. Negative attitudes and perceptions about sleep take hold. A rigorous review of sleep hygiene can ease the distress felt by many patients in the grip of chronic insomnia.

It must be stressed that insomnia is much more a waking disorder than a sleeping disorder. In fact, insomniac patients appear to have hyperactive waking mechanisms, especially at bedtime. As well, they experience a less significant drop in the brain metabolism associated with slow wave sleep, particularly in regions such as the hypothalamus and brain stem, where the wake and sleep centres are located. The brains of these people are therefore more active during sleep than are those of sleepers who do not have insomnia.

HOW CAN YOU TELL HOW SERIOUS YOUR INSOMNIA IS?

The severity of insomnia is determined by the degree of disruption it causes in patients' lives. When people who normally should sleep seven to nine hours a night start sleeping fewer than six and a half hours, they are deemed to have insomnia. In chronic insomnia disorders, people take more than thirty minutes to fall asleep more than three times a week, over a period of six consecutive months. This is, however, only an average used to assess the sleep habits and individual needs of each patient.

To determine whether patients are natural short sleepers or insomniacs, a doctor checks to see if they feel any nega-

CONDITIONS THAT CAN CAUSE INSOMNIA

Insomnia is not considered a diagnosis in itself, but rather the expression of an underlying problem.

Sleep disorder

Chronic psychophysiological insomnia	Insomnia associated with an elevated level of muscle and psychological tension at night. Its symptoms are difficulty falling asleep, waking up in the night, non-restorative sleep, and daytime fatigue.
Periodic leg movements during sleep and restless legs syndrome	Difficulty falling asleep, along with a tingling sensation in the legs. Sleep disrupted at night by leg movements.
Sleep apnea	Sleep apnea disorder often leads to daytime drowsiness. Many patients also experience nighttime sleep disrupted by respiratory pauses.
Circadian rhythm disorders	Sleep schedule disorders with insomnia at times when sleep is desired. The insomnia symptoms generally include difficulty falling asleep or waking up too early in the morning.

Psychological/psychiatric condition

Stress, anxiety	Difficulty falling asleep, nighttime awakenings, non-restorative sleep.
Depression	Insomnia, often accompanied by waking up too early in the morning and feeling sad in the morning.
Bipolar affective disorder	Insomnia, reduced need of sleep and excessive energy in the hypomanic and manic phases.
Post-traumatic stress disorder	Disrupted nighttime sleep and nightmares.
Premenstrual dysphoric disorder	Insomnia or hypersomnia.
Schizophrenia	Sleep schedule often out of sync, lighter and less restorative sleep.

Medical condition

Gastroesophageal reflux	Sleep disrupted by the reflux and daytime fatigue.
Asthma	Sleep disrupted by nighttime asthma attacks.
Heart failure	Breathing and sleep disrupted by lying on the back.
Arthritis and other medical conditions causing nighttime pain	Sleep disrupted by pain.
Neurological disorders (stroke, Alzheimer's disease, Parkinson's disease, multiple sclerosis)	Nighttime restlessness, schedule and sleep disrupted.

FIGURE 19

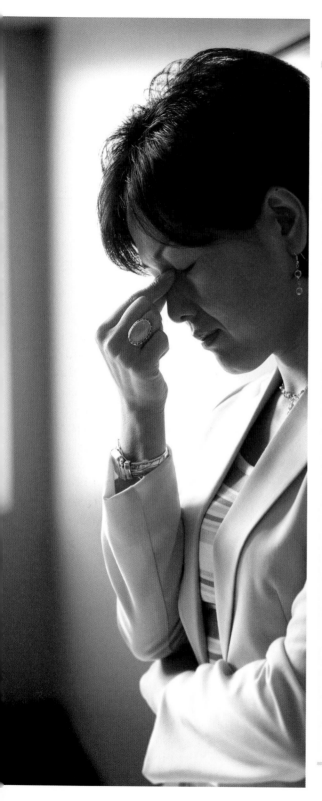

DAYTIME SYMPTOMS OF SLEEP DEPRIVATION

Sleep deprivation can cause various kinds of psychological and physical distress. Symptoms will vary depending on how serious the sleep deprivation is and how well a person tolerates it. The first symptoms to appear are usually psychological.

Psychological symptoms

- Irritability, aggressiveness
- Social withdrawal
- Sadness
- Decrease in libido

Cognitive problems

- Diminished mental faculties and acuity
- Difficulties concentrating
- Memory impairment
- Learning difficulties
- Decreased creativity
- Confusion

Physical ailments

- Fatigue, drowsiness
- Nausea, loss of appetite
- Dizziness
- Migraines
- Feeling cold, sweating
- Muscle coordination problems
- Impaired reflexes
- Vision blurred
- Heart palpitations
- Hormonal disturbances

FIGURE 20

tive impacts from sleep deprivation. Lack of sleep leads to fatigue and a myriad of ailments the next day, affecting patients' moods, intellectual abilities, and physical performance (Figure 20). Fatigue and drowsiness are reported during the day, which increases the risk of being the victim of a workplace or car accident. Patients' moods are also affected by sleep debt and they often experience anxiety, sadness, irritability, and even depression. They may report memory disorders, difficulty concentrating, and less intellectual creativity. Insomnia thus causes a great deal of individual distress and has significant negative impacts on the quality of professional, family, and social lives.

PREDISPOSING FACTORS FOR INSOMNIA

There are several predisposing risk factors for insomnia, the most important being age and sex. Complaints of insomnia are more common in the elderly: approximately 15 to 50 percent of the elderly population appears to be affected. In young adults, problems getting to sleep are more common, while older people mainly have difficulty staying asleep. These different kinds of insomnia depending on age category correspond to changes in the sleep-wake cycle that occur naturally over a lifetime. As we have seen, adolescents tend to have a timetable out of sync with the general population, naturally going to bed and getting up later. Once out of this stage, a large number of young adults maintain this tendency to the point where their sleep schedule becomes a problem in their academic and professional lives. In young adults, serious problems falling asleep, combined with difficulty getting up, fatigue, and morning drowsiness, are a sign of a circadian rhythm disorder called delayed sleep phase disorder. The circadian rhythms of body temperature and melatonin secretion in these young people are several hours off, in comparison with good sleepers of the same age. In contrast, with age, circadian rhythms and sleep schedules have a tendency to shift to an earlier time of day. When this trend is taken to extremes, people may fall asleep and naturally wake up earlier than they want to, and even suffer from early morning awakening.

Elderly patients are more likely to develop the circadian rhythm disorder known as advanced sleep phase disorder, a condition rarely seen in people under forty. That said, sleep changes that go along with aging are more complex than a simple exaggerated tendency to become a morning person. In cases of advanced sleep phase disorder, the circadian rhythms of body temperature and melatonin secretion occur several hours earlier than in good sleepers of the same age. Note that we must be careful not to confuse this particular disorder with depression, another condition in which early morning awakening occurs.

Women are twice as likely as men to have insomnia. Differences in exposure to sex hormones (estrogens, progesterone, and testosterone) might be involved.

Patients with psychological and psychiatric disorders, such as depression, bipolar affective disorder, chronic anxiety, premenstrual dysphoric disorder, and schizophrenia, are also at risk. These illnesses are described in greater detail in Chapter 6.

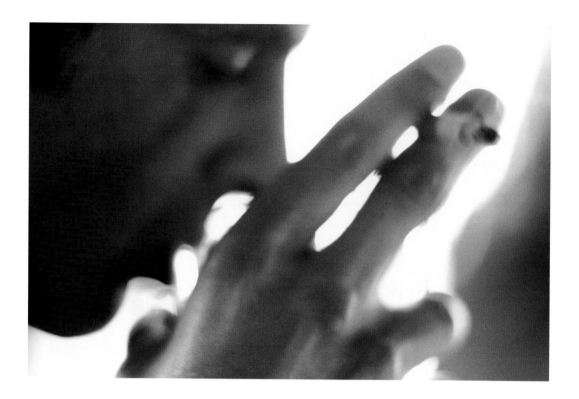

People with poor lifestyle habits — excessive consumption of alcohol, caffeinated beverages, street drugs — are also at higher risk. Drinking a few glasses of wine or a few beers in the evening may help you fall asleep, but the sleep that ensues is often of poorer quality, restless, and shorter, especially if large amounts have been consumed. Caffeine counteracts the effect of adenosine receptors, a neurotransmitter that promotes sleep. Drinking coffee, tea, or energy drinks in the morning can help fight fatigue. On the other hand, in the afternoon and evening, these substances are likely to keep you from falling asleep. Limiting their consumption and avoiding them after lunch is strongly recommended. Street drugs like ecstasy have a very pronounced and disruptive effect on the internal organization of sleep.

Several chronic diseases increase the risk of insomnia. This is the case with diseases like asthma, whose symptoms get worse during the night. There are also diseases that make it harder to remain lying down; these include heart failure, owing to the pulmonary congestion that the prone position causes, and gastro-esophageal reflux, since the reflux and burning sensations are stronger when lying down, especially when people go to bed on a full stomach. A number of health problems also disrupt sleep, one example being arthritis, which wakes patients up at night because of the pain. In other cases, some medications given to treat patients can disrupt sleep. This is called iatrogenic insomnia, in other words, insomnia related to medical treatment.

The list of substances that interfere with sleep is a long one, and insomnia is among

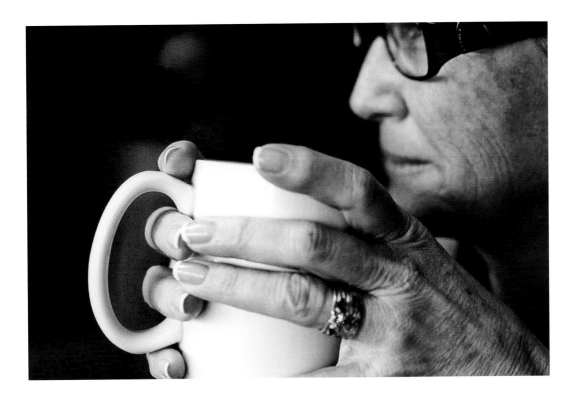

the side effects caused by many medications, a few of which are listed in Figure 21. Debilitating illnesses should also be mentioned, particularly neurological disorders like strokes, Parkinson's disease, multiple sclerosis or Alzheimer's disease, which are sometimes accompanied by a disorganized sleep-wake cycle.

It should be stressed that insomnia is a complaint that may be associated with other sleep disorders; before confirming so-called chronic psychophysiological insomnia a doctor will be sure to screen carefully for other illnesses that can cause the insomnia, such as sleep apnea or restless legs syndrome. These disorders will be described in more detail in Chapters 8 and 9.

When insomnia involves a disruption in the alternation between periods of sleeping and waking, we are dealing with circadian rhythm disorders. As we saw in Chapter 2, these include difficulties in adjusting to nighttime work, jet lag, delayed and advanced sleep phase disorders, a non-twenty-four- hour sleep disorder, and an irregular sleep-wake schedule.

INSOMNIA'S LONG-TERM IMPACTS

It is now clear that persistent insomnia is associated with an elevated risk of falling prey to many health problems, especially mental health disorders (Chapter 6). In 40 percent of cases, insomnia precedes the onset of severe depression by several years, but the relationship between insomnia and mental health is usually bi-directional. In other words, sleep disruptions increase the likelihood of developing a mental health disorder, and mental illnesses are usually

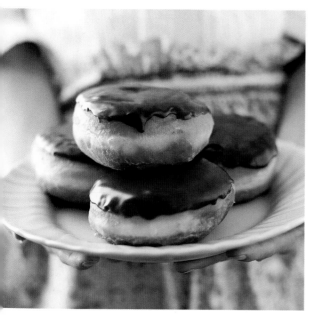

SLEEP-DISRUPTING MEDICATIONS AND SUBSTANCES

Foods, over-the-counter drugs, and street drugs

- Caffeine, tea, energy drinks
- Chocolate
- Alcohol
- Decongestants, cold pills
- Tobacco
- Cocaine
- Ecstasy

Prescription drugs

- Some antidepressants
- Some painkillers
- Prolonged daily use of sleeping pills*
- Steroids
- Synthroid (levothyroxine)
- Psychostimulants like dextroamphetamine (Dexedrine), methylphenidate (Ritalin), and modafinil (Alertec)
- Antiparkinsonian drugs
- Nicotine patches

Not an exhaustive list. Sleep disruptions depend on the dose of the substance ingested and the period of ingestion. They also vary from person to person.

*Paradoxically, sleeping pills can aggravate an insomnia problem by disrupting the structure of sleep and causing rebound insomnia when they are suddenly stopped. This is why it's advisable to plan to stop taking them gradually.

FIGURE 21

linked to sleep disorders. The sleep disorders associated with psychiatric illnesses are often serious and resist treatment, making caring for the patient more complicated (Buysse et al., 2008). Like the chicken and the egg, which comes first: sleep disorders or mental illness?

Patients with insomnia call on health services more often than good sleepers, since physical health can be affected by sleep schedule disruptions. Disruptions in the metabolism of sugars and fats and in appetite control are front and centre. The expression "they who sleep forget their hunger" has never been more pertinent, now that the scientific community is actively exploring the connections between sleep, diet, and excess weight. Missing out on a few hours of sleep every day can affect the metabolism of sugars and create a state comparable to that of a patient with pre-diabetes. After a poor night's sleep, the levels of sugar in the blood rise higher when high-sugar foods are eaten than they do after a good night.

This indicates that the body develops a temporary resistance to the effect of insulin after not having slept for a few hours. The metabolic impacts of sleep disruptions will be discussed in greater detail in Chapter 5.

Sleep disruptions may also be associated with decreased control over blood pressure in hypertensive patients. In healthy people, blood pressure fluctuates during the day and drops by 10 to 20 percent during sleep. In hypertensive patients this rhythm often fluctuates abnormally, a problem that sleep disruptions can aggravate.

ADVICE FOR SLEEPING WELL

When insomnia is a problem, it's important to establish good sleep hygiene. In fact, it's useful in any sleep disorder to review behaviours associated with waking and sleeping times. The overall goal of good sleep hygiene is to help us fall asleep quickly and get efficient and restorative sleep, waking up in the night as little as possible after we have gone to sleep. Since insomnia is more a waking problem than a sleeping problem, several pieces of advice in Figure 22 focus on reducing mental and physical hyperactivity at bedtime. Factors making mental and physical tension worse at bedtime must be minimized. It's important, for example, to allow yourself a period of transition at the end of the evening to relax. During this period, you must stop working or playing on the Internet right up to the last minute, avoid intense sports late in the evening, and not watch TV or answer emails in bed.

Making a point of hiding the clock is an essential piece of advice. You must at all costs resist the desire to know what time it is when you can't sleep at night. Merely looking at the time triggers a series of negative thoughts that only make sleep concerns worse. Even people who think they are immune to insomnia have a tendency to mentally calculate the rest they've accumulated during the night up to that point and the number of hours they have left to sleep. But the recovery component of nighttime sleep cannot be calculated that easily. The equation is more complex and follows instead an inverse exponential function, and even that is too simple. We therefore need to let our unconscious brain do the calculation on its own and give our neurons a rest. The alarm clock should be set to go off at the right time, but you must not look at the time during the night or in the early morning.

Other pieces of advice on sleep hygiene aim to promote good quality sleep. For example, insomniac patients should do all they can to maximize their sleep pressure (the homeostatic process). For this reason they must avoid naps during the day, since they lower sleep pressure. In the morning they have to avoid staying in bed too long, since by doing so the process of fatigue accumulation during the day is delayed. As a consequence, this would make falling asleep in the evening more difficult. Patients must therefore observe their chosen wake-up time.

Since the biological clock strongly influences an individual's ability to fall asleep, patients should also maintain sleep habits that promote good synchronization between their sleep times and their biological clock. This is why keeping wake times and bedtimes as regular as possible is recommended, even on days off. While going

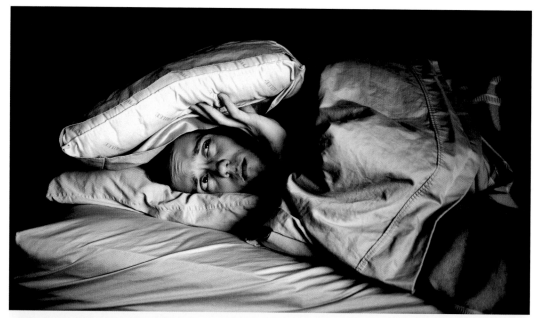

Dr. Ivan Pavlov and You

Pavlov's experiment with dogs is famous and clearly illustrates what we call a conditioned reflex. During this experiment, the researcher systematically offered food to a dog after having exposed it to the sound of a whistle, tuning fork or metronome. The dog salivated on seeing the food. Quite quickly, just hearing the noise caused the dog to salivate automatically, since the noise indicated that food was going to appear in its dish. The dog had unconsciously associated what was for it an unimportant event (the sound of the whistle) with another emotionally important one (the arrival of food). This salivation reflex is a conditioned response, since it's induced by a neutral stimulus (the sound of the whistle) associated with a stimulus that triggers an unconscious reaction (the presence of food). In the absence of food, this conditioned reflex becomes inappropriate.

A similar situation occurs in the case of chronic insomnia. Insomniac patients often stay in bed in their room for many hours, wide awake, in the hope of getting a few hours of sleep. In so doing, they wrongly think they are increasing their chances of falling asleep. But, quite quickly, their brain associates their bedroom with staying awake. What's more, by this time they are often in a state of frustration and mental hyperactivity, with ideas rushing around in their head, muscle tension and negative thoughts. If in addition they have the bad idea of looking at the clock, this state of mental and physical tension only gets worse as the night goes on.

Unfortunately, Pavlov's experiment proves to be true, and their brain associates their bedroom with a state of wakefulness and mental hyperactivity.

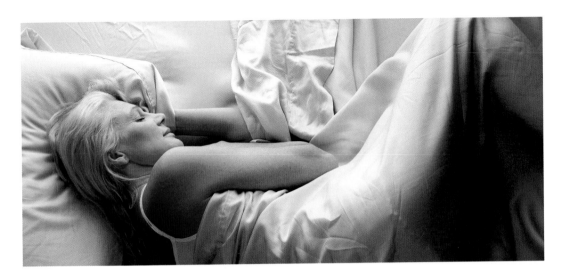

THE INSOMNIAC'S TEN COMMANDMENTS

These pieces of advice are important elements of good sleep hygiene and are suggested for patients with insomnia.

1. Keep your sleep times as regular as possible. First establish your wake time and go to bed in the evening when you feel the need to sleep. Your sleep times will gradually adjust.

2. Keep your exposure times to light and dark as regular as possible. Get as much sunlight as you can during the day. Sleep in the dark and remain in dim light at night if you get out of bed.

3. Relax but avoid napping if you feel very tired during the day.

4. Avoid using alcohol or drugs to help you sleep.

5. Leave your bedroom if you wake up at night and have difficulty getting back to sleep. Relax in dim light in another room until you feel the need to go back to sleep. Avoid stimulating activities (housework, work, email, Internet) in the middle of the night.

6. Resist at all costs the desire to look at the clock at night! Set your alarm to go off at your desired regular wake time.

7. Avoid consuming too many stimulating substances during the day (except for medical prescriptions).

8. Only use your bedroom for sleeping (and sexual activity). Banish work, TV, iPad, cell phones, and any other stimulating activity from it.

9. Sleep in a calm, dark, comfortably cool and well-ventilated environment.

10. Plan a time for rest and leisure every day, especially in the evening.

FIGURE 22   Adapted from Diane B. Boivin, "Docteur, je ne dors pas!" Information module, Fédération des médecins omnipraticiens du Québec (Quebec federation of general practitioners), Montreal, 1993.

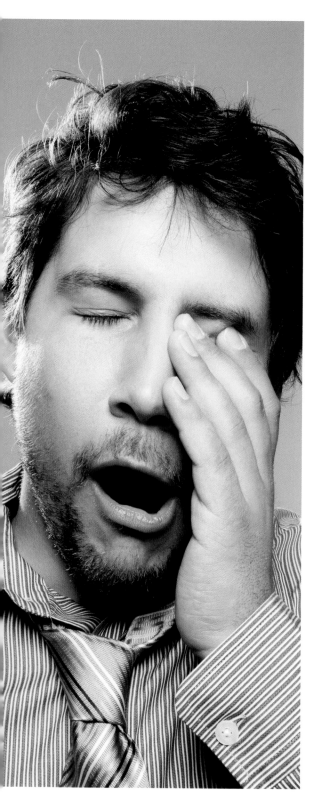

to bed too late is not good, going to bed too early must also be avoided; otherwise, bedtime coincides with the time when the biological clock is sending its strongest wake-up signals. This period of the evening is called "the forbidden zone for sleep" and occurs one or two hours before normal bedtime (Strogatz et al., 1987). As small a difference as one or two hours in our sleep schedule can thus have a marked impact on our quality of sleep and our waking period.

This is in fact what we experience in autumn and spring when we switch to standard time and to daylight saving time, respectively. Some people are very sensitive to these changes and can sometimes take a week to get used to them. What's more, in the spring these adjustments include sleep deprivation, since our sleep is shortened by an hour compared with standard time. In the autumn, the time change is accompanied by an extra hour of sleep, which is better for recovering from fatigue. On the other hand, there is less light in the environment in the autumn, and this increases many people's fatigue levels.

Other methods should also be tried. For example, to ensure your biological clock is aligned correctly with your environment, you should not be exposed to intense light late at night or in the middle of the night, as this can cause the circadian clock to shift to a later time, and even trigger delayed phase disorder or reduce the secretion of melatonin at night.

HOW CAN YOU CURE YOUR INSOMNIA?

We should first specify that you should not try to *cure* your insomnia, but instead learn to minimize its impacts. Wanting at any cost to get a normal or even perfect sleep every single night only makes the tensions and worries linked to insomnia worse. It's a little like wanting to cure anxiety by forcing yourself, whatever the cost, to relax. It's much better to let go and learn to put your expectations about sleep into perspective. This message may seem contradictory: on the one hand, we are told about the mental and physical health risks of disrupted sleep and on the other we are told not to pay too much attention to it. In fact, what we really have to tackle is the performance anxiety associated with sleep. The good news is that insomnia rarely kills, and that even though it damages physical and mental health, this process occurs very slowly. Cases of fatal familial insomnia are extremely rare (the author of this book has never come across a single one in her twenty-five year career).

Since it's completely normal for sleep to become more fragile with age, patients have to set realistic goals. It's wiser to re-examine your perceptions about sleep, especially since many insomniacs tend to underestimate the length of time they sleep at night. It's therefore important for patients to cultivate a degree of detachment with regard to their insomnia. Insomnia is in fact a chronic condition that has settled in for the long haul. You have to expect that it will take a long time to regain a better quality sleep.

Even after you've tried to improve your sleep hygiene, you still may not be rid of your insomnia. Various non-pharmacological strategies should then be considered to reduce it. One of these approaches is to tackle the conditioned reflex. This is called a stimulus control approach and it tries to lower the risks of associating the bedroom with not sleeping. In this approach, when patients

reach a state of frustration at not being able to sleep, they are instructed to relax in a different room. Only light activities that make you feel like you want to go back to sleep, like reading, listening to relaxing music, or practicing relaxation techniques, should be engaged in. Activities that are too stimulating must be avoided, such as answering emails, instant messaging, playing video games, or, even worse, working. When the need to sleep gets stronger, patients are encouraged to return to their bedroom to sleep. This process is to be repeated as often as necessary.

Sleep restriction is another approach that aims to improve sleep efficiency by imposing tight control over the times when sleeping is permitted (Taylor et al., 2010). The goal of this approach is to keep you from spending long periods of

IMOVANE (ZOPICLONE)

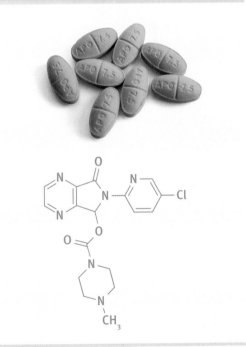

FIGURE 23

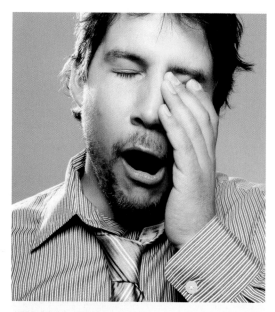

Did You Yawn?

Experiments have been done with humans, baboons, and dogs to try to understand why yawning is contagious (Palagi et al., 2009). Neurologically, the act of yawning seems to raise vigilance levels. Animals may use yawning as a means of social communication to inform their fellow creatures about their level of fatigue and stress. This means of communication would thus enable a group of animals to synchronize their active and resting rhythms. Yawning is also contagious in humans and a good 50 percent of us seem to yawn after having seen, heard or merely thought of another person who is yawning. If you gave in to the temptation when you saw the picture above, don't worry, heightened sensitivity to contagious yawning goes along with a higher level of empathy. So don't get discouraged if one day your doctor yawns in your face...

time in your bedroom without sleeping. For example, patients who say they only sleep four hours a night, but spend eight hours lying in bed trying to sleep, have a sleep efficiency of roughly 50 percent. Patients are instructed to limit the time they spend in bed to four hours a night and to avoid daytime naps so as to maximize their homeostatic sleep pressure. Their sleep efficiency then rises quickly to nearly 100 percent. Since this is quite a radical sleep regimen, it's a temporary measure. The "sleep ratio" will in fact be increased little by little, by several minutes a day, until a period of sleep of acceptable quality and length is achieved.

In chronic psychophysiological insomnia (insomnia not explained by another disease), there is a great deal of anxiety and worry about sleep. Relaxation therapies have proven very useful in the long-term treatment of this kind of insomnia (McKinstry et al., 2008).

We have described here the biological bases of sleep and chronic insomnia. The most severe cases of insomnia may need medical treatment. This treatment will involve the controlled use of sleeping pills as well as learning relaxation therapies. In all cases of insomnia, it's important to review sleep hygiene. The advice given in this chapter will help those suffering from insomnia to re-examine their lifestyle habits in order to minimize the consequences.

What Should You Take Away From This Chapter?

- Insomnia differs from natural short sleep in that sufferers experience unpleasant symptoms during the day. These psychological and physical symptoms are indicative of sleep deprivation.

- Insomnia is much more a waking disorder than a sleeping disorder. Mental hyperactivity and muscle tension occur when a patient tries unsuccessfully to sleep.

- Insomnia is a symptom that manifests itself as a recurring difficulty in falling asleep or staying asleep. Several sleep disorders, medical conditions, or substances can cause or maintain this problem, and they must be identified if they are to be controlled.

- Most of the time, an insomnia problem begins suddenly after a difficult life situation. A chronic sleep problem can persist on its own.

- There are several pieces of advice patients can take to promote sound sleep. This advice aims to maximize sleep pressure at night and make sure the sleep schedule and the biological clock are in harmony.

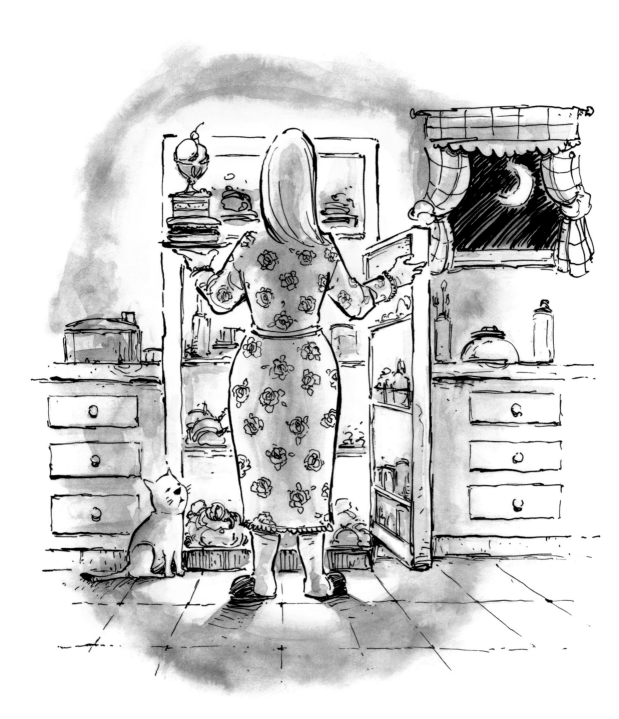

Why sleep when you can eat?

CHAPTER 5

They Who Sleep Forget Their Hunger!

Sleep and Diet

Several epidemiological studies carried out in various countries have confirmed the disturbing and worsening problem of obesity in modern society. At the same time, other studies show a gradual decline in hours of sleep at night, especially during the work week. There appears to be a connection therefore between lack of sleep and obesity (Magee et al., 2010). Studies indicate that the daily quality and quantity of sleep affect eating patterns, food metabolism, and the risk of becoming overweight, even in children (Figure 24).

These observations are not surprising, given the key role sleep plays in energy conservation. This conservation depends on a drop in metabolism at night and on biological changes that cause the body to rest and not feel hungry. Several key dietary and metabolic hormones, like leptin, ghrelin, and insulin, also act on maintenance of wakefulness and maintenance of sleep systems. The level of these hormones is influenced by the length of sleep episodes and their schedule. The loss of a few hours of sleep a night or a sudden change in sleep schedule causes metabolic disruptions that need to be looked at closely. Many people face this situation regularly, including patients with sleep disorders and nighttime workers. The relationships between sleep, energy conservation, recovery, metabolism, and diet will be discussed in this chapter.

SLEEP AND BRAIN RECOVERY

During the night, our bodies go into energy conservation mode. Energy needs fall because we expend much less energy during the night than during the day. In slow wave sleep, oxygen and glucose metabolism and the flow of blood to the brain are 25 to 40 percent below levels seen in the waking period. This decline in energy needs can be partially explained by the fact we are lying down and therefore no longer use muscle energy to maintain a standing position. Our physical activities are also greatly reduced during sleep. However, the decrease in energy consumption is not explained only by the fact that we stop performing the physical and mental activities we do while awake. In fact, our brain itself consumes less energy when we sleep than when we are awake. During nocturnal sleep, the slowdown in brain metabolism is responsible for two-thirds of the decline in the organism's glucose consumption. In general, it can be said that the brain also goes into energy conservation mode during sleep, especially during slow wave sleep. This is important if we are to recover from the neuronal fatigue accumulated during the preceding waking period. Experimental

evidence indicates that neurons communicate intensely among themselves during waking periods, and that at the end of the day the neuronal communication systems, called synapses, are used even more actively, which could cause excessive energy demands if the situation were to continue. Fortunately, during sleep, these connections lose some of their strength, which lets us start the new day able to prioritize the communications among neurons that meet our new intellectual and physical needs (Olcese et al., 2010). The remodelling of the strength of neuronal connections is clear evidence of what is called "nervous system plasticity" — its tremendous adaptability.

A slowdown in brain metabolism has been shown to occur during slow wave sleep in the brain stem, thalamus, and several regions of the cerebral cortex (Dang-Vu et al., 2010). It's interesting to note that the brain regions most in use

TV WATCHING, SLEEP, AND OBESITY

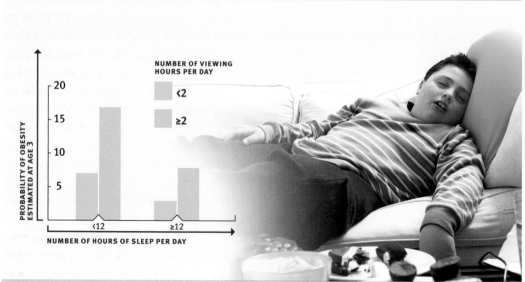

FIGURE 24

Adapted from Taveras et al., 2008.

when we are awake, such as the frontal and parietal regions involved in high-level brain activities, seem to have the greatest need for recovery. A noticeable slowdown in brain metabolism is indeed seen in these regions during slow wave sleep. Even when sleep deprivation is imposed on the organism, it has been observed that the metabolism in these frontal regions of the cerebral cortex drops, and there is an overall slowdown in brain metabolism.

In addition, these observations have been correlated with the weakening of cognitive abilities and judgment typical of extreme sleep deprivation. Furthermore, the brain regions that play a major role in generating slow EEG waves and sleep spindles are activated during sleep.

In patients with chronic insomnia, the brain metabolism associated with slow wave sleep slows down less, especially in regions like the hypothalamus and brain stem, where the wake and sleep centres are located. This observation is a reminder that insomnia is first and foremost a disorder caused by hyperactive wakefulness-promoting mechanisms.

In comparison, energy needs during REM sleep, the stage of sleep typically associated with dreams, are much closer to waking needs, even though the active and less active brain areas are different in these two states of consciousness. The brain regions most active during REM sleep are precisely those involved in causing rapid eye movements (REM, and the ponto-geniculo-occipital waves preceding these movements) — the pontine tegmentum, the lateral geniculate bodies and the occipital cortex.

SLEEP AND PHYSICAL RECOVERY

At bedtime in the evening, the simple fact of lying down in the dark, calm and relaxed, triggers a series of physiological reactions that allow the body gradually to drift off to sleep (Boudreau et al., 2012). The more tonic mechanisms that predominate when we are awake gradually make way for those that promote sleep. Thus, the transition from waking to sleeping is accompanied by a change in the activation of the cardiovascular and respiratory systems, brought about by what's called the autonomic nervous system.

During our waking periods, the tone of the autonomic nervous system is mainly sympathetic. In contrast, during periods of slow wave sleep, the tone of the autonomic nervous system is mainly parasympathetic. The pulse, for example, is faster when we are awake during the day than when we are asleep at night. As soon as we fall asleep, the heart slows down and the interval between heartbeats gets roughly 10 percent longer compared with what is observed during waking periods. This slowdown in heart rate reaches its peak in the phases of slow wave sleep. The transition from sleeping to waking when we get up in the morning is accompanied by a faster irregular heartbeat. These sleep-related pulse fluctuations are also intensified by the influence of the biological clock. Heart rate thus varies in accordance with internal biological time, slowing down at night and speeding up during the day. In other words, sleep has a calming effect on the heart.

Blood pressure also fluctuates during the day. It increases in the morning in the hours after we get up and reaches its peak in the afternoon. Blood pressure begins

The Autonomic Nervous System

The autonomic nervous system automatically regulates, without our making any conscious efforts, the heart, blood vessels, and respiratory and digestive systems. This is the system that speeds up the heartbeat, causes blood pressure to rise, and makes breathing deeper and faster when an individual is in a stressful situation, or perhaps faces potential danger. This same system also activates the digestive system and redirects blood toward it after a meal.

The autonomic nervous system is divided into the sympathetic and parasympathetic nervous systems. These two systems, like yin and yang, have opposite but complementary effects on the organism. The sympathetic system stimulates more pronounced activity, while the parasympathetic system induces a more relaxed vegetative state. Although the autonomic nervous system is regulated automatically, it can be modulated by conscious activities like meditation and relaxation, which have the effect of slowing heart rate, respiratory rate, and, in the most experienced, blood pressure.

Awakening is accompanied by increased sympathetic tone and decreased parasympathetic tone. The opposite occurs during sleep, especially deep sleep.

to drop again in the evening and reaches its lowest point in the middle of the night. Heart rate and blood pressure reach their lowest daily level during slow wave sleep.

During REM sleep, the pulse and blood pressure reach levels much closer to those seen during wakefulness, but are very irregular. The activation of the autonomic nervous system becomes erratic during phases of dreaming.

The circadian rhythm of melatonin secretion could be a factor in increasing sleep-related blood pressure fluctuations. Melatonin can indeed cause a drop in blood pressure; a number of studies have shown that a deficiency in the secretion of this hormone may be linked to high blood pressure. These observations illustrate the beneficial effects of nighttime sleep, especially slow wave sleep, on the cardiovascular system. The noticeable fluctuations in cardiovascular functions related to the sleep-wake cycle and circadian system might contribute to the increased risk of cardiovascular events reported in the early hours of the morning. A 40 percent increase in the risk of myocardial infarction and a 30 percent increase in the risk of sudden death in the morning compared with the rest of the day have in fact been observed.

The respiratory system also undergoes significant changes during sleep. These will be described in Chapter 8, which deals with respiratory problems during sleep.

SLEEP, BODY TEMPERATURE, AND ENERGY CONSERVATION

Body temperature is the result of the production and dissipation of heat by the body. It fluctuates greatly during the day. Generally, core body temperature, measured using a rectal thermometer, ranges from 36.75 to 37.5 degrees Celsius. The temperature measured on the surface of the skin of the arms and legs is lower, at around 32.5 to 34 degrees Celsius. Changes in body temperature tell us about the human body's energy consumption. It's important to keep body temperature as stable as possible, within a fairly restricted comfort zone, in order to be able to survive. In fact, body temperature ultimately influences the quality of the biological activities and chemical reactions that occur in every cell in the human body. As proof, we just have to recall the meteorological alerts issued by Health Canada during summer heat waves or severe winter cold spells.

The body's heat production depends on food intake and metabolism, ensuring that nutrients reach the cells where they can be used. Calories (from the Latin *calor*, "heat") are used as a unit of measure to quantify the energy value of a food. Body heat dissipates when we burn calories; the heat produced by the body is then released into the environment. This heat dissipation increases during intense physical activity, as we are burning more calories than usual. Food is therefore a kind of wood or heating oil for the human body.

Because of this thermal energy, a rheostatic system is needed to control temperature levels throughout the body. This system has a central unit, somewhat like a furnace and its control panel, located in the hypothalamus, right in the middle of the brain. It also has a peripheral control system in the skin, especially at the ends of the legs and arms. The central control system determines the threshold at which the body should take action to conserve or dissipate heat. The peripheral control system in turn is very efficient at retaining heat or releasing it into the environment, somewhat as if we opened many windows when body temperature was too high, or the opposite. The peripheral control system is mainly composed of a great many arteriovenous anastomoses, which are the extreme ends of the vascular tree in the peripheral tissues (Chapter 8).

Significant fluctuations in body temperature occur during the day, influenced by the circadian system and the sleep-wake cycle. This observation is not surprising, as the preoptic area of the anterior hypothalamus is the main control centre for sleep and body temperature. At bedtime, the body, trying to conserve its energy and recover as much as possible during nighttime sleep, sets its rheostats to maintain a central body temperature that is lower than during the waking period. A cascade of events then takes place at bedtime. Vascular dilation is first noticed in the arms and legs. Many arteriovenous anastomoses dilate in the fingers and toes, allowing heat to dissipate quickly and efficiently (as if we opened the windows after overheating). This process is aided by the relaxation that accompanies a decrease in the tone of the sympathetic nervous system, as well as the secretion of melatonin in the evening. The latter in fact promotes dilation of the arteriovenous anastomoses late in the evening and hence the dissipation of body heat. Hands and feet thus get warmer at bedtime, so much so that it helps put us to sleep quickly and efficiently. As the heat dissipates into the environment via the hands and feet, internal body temperature drops. This cooling system lets the body

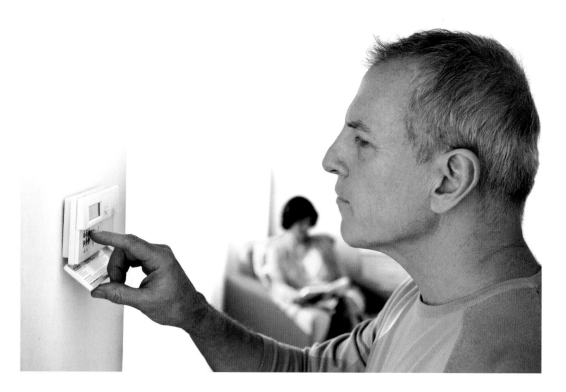

function with a lower energy level, as if there were fewer logs in the woodstove at night during sleep. Core body temperature reaches its lowest point at the end of the night, approximately one or two hours before normal wake time.

Body temperature changes observed during sleep make the sleeper more sensitive to environmental temperature fluctuations. To sleep well, therefore, it's important to control bedroom temperature and avoid room temperatures that are either too hot or too cold. Brain temperature also drops during sleep, especially during slow wave sleep. On the other hand, it remains high during REM sleep, a reminder that this stage of sleep is different and involves a state of heightened cortical activity while we dream.

THE DIGESTIVE SYSTEM DURING THE SLEEP-WAKE CYCLE

The functioning of the digestive system also changes significantly during the sleep-wake cycle. To understand these changes, a review of the anatomy of this system and how it works may be useful (Figure 25). The digestive system begins in the mouth, the organism's entry point for food, and ends at the anus, the exit point for food that has been digested but not absorbed. Between the two, there is an entire factory for decomposing and absorbing food, an overview of which is outside the scope of this book. Nonetheless, it's helpful to be familiar with certain aspects of this system that can influence the quality of nighttime sleep.

When food is ingested, it's initially broken down in the stomach, where highly acidic gastric juices go to work tenderizing it. The stomach is really a biological bag where food is mixed with gastric juices. When we are awake, food intake triggers the production of these gastric juices and the "food-demolition" factory starts up. During sleep, however, a circadian rhythm regulates stomach acidity level. This rhythm causes the acidity to reach its peak late in the evening and early in the night. It's therefore very important for the stomach to empty properly at that time and for its contents to move in the right direction — downward into the duodenum and not upward to the esophagus. The lower esophageal sphincter helps keep the gastric contents in the stomach; its tonus decreases during sleep, compared with when we are awake, a situation which can hinder the emptying of the stomach in the right direction. What's more, saliva production and the swallowing reflex, important processes for neutralizing gastric acidity, decrease sharply during sleep. The sleep period is therefore risky for patients with digestive disorders.

The movement of gastric contents upward into the esophagus is called gastroesophageal reflux. It can be very irritating for the esophagus and cause unpleasant burning sensations. In the most serious cases, the mucus membrane of the esophagus can be greatly inflamed, a condition called esophagitis. When gastroesophageal reflux occurs during sleep, it takes longer for the corrosive liquid to return to the stomach because of the altered state of consciousness. It can easily take twice as long during sleep as in the waking period.

Episodes of nighttime reflux can also cause respiratory symptoms such as asthma attacks during the night. Nearly one in two

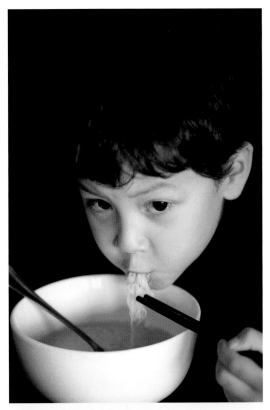

Hunger and Satiety Hormones

Leptin is a satiety hormone produced by adipose cells (adipocytes). Its levels decrease when the body needs food and increase when it's full. Ghrelin is a hunger hormone produced by the gastric mucosa. Its levels increase before every meal and drop again in the hours afterward. These two hormones thus have a reciprocal effect on appetite.

patients with a gastroesophageal reflux problem complains of sleep disruptions caused by nighttime reflux. It's therefore important not to go to bed on a full stomach and to avoid alcohol and spicy foods in the evening. Furthermore, sleeping in the left lateral decubitus position (on the left side) rather than in the dorsal decubitus position (on the back) can facilitate the emptying of the stomach. Patients with a duodenal gastric ulcer also experience a recurrence of their burning sensations at night. Taking antacids during the evening can help reduce these irritations, but medical treatment is recommended in the case of persistent problems.

Once through the stomach, the semi-digested food travels through the other parts of the digestive tract. It's interesting to note that the distension of certain parts of the intestine can cause drowsiness. As food passes through the intestine, this may also stimulate the secretion of intestinal hormones, such as cholecystokinin or bombesin, or the pancreatic hormone, insulin. Studies show that these hormones may have a hypnogenic effect (which promotes sleep). In

THE DIGESTIVE SYSTEM

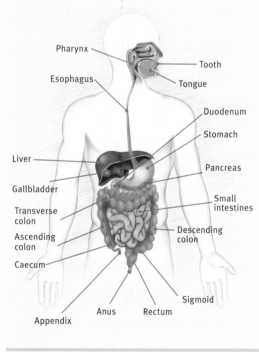

Pharynx
Tooth
Esophagus
Tongue
Duodenum
Stomach
Liver
Pancreas
Gallbladder
Small intestines
Transverse colon
Ascending colon
Descending colon
Caecum
Sigmoid
Anus   Rectum
Appendix

FIGURE 25

addition, leptin, a satiety hormone produced by adipose cells after a meal, counteracts the arousing effect of the orexin/hypocretin system described in Chapter 1. It's possible, therefore, that the production of substances closely associated with diet may help make some people drowsy after a good meal....

SLEEP AND DIET

Our body is made to expect to be deprived of food for about eight hours, or during a night's sleep. As a result, not eating while sleeping is not a problem; as they say, "They who sleep forget their hunger!" There is no danger at all in terms of energy, since metabolic needs are reduced during sleep. Glycemic levels (the levels of blood sugar or glucose in the blood) actually remain quite constant during a night's sleep, even though food intake is interrupted. This is because nocturnal metabolism slows down and cells have less access to blood glucose. In effect, the organism keeps its glucose in the blood longer. The result of the body's adaptation to "temporary nightly starvation" is that it does not respond well when mealtimes are suddenly changed. In fact, the body metabolizes food differently if it's ingested at night instead of during the day.

When blood sugar rises in the blood after a meal, the pancreas secretes insulin so that glucose can enter the cells, where it will be used. This process then lowers blood sugar. A meal rich in carbohydrates — for example bread, pasta, etc. — causes a more dramatic rise in blood sugar and insulin if it's eaten in the early hours of the night instead of in the morning! This indicates that temporary resistance to the effect of insulin has occurred. These changes are similar to what is considered to be a state of risk for developing diabetes. Similarly, a meal rich in fats will cause a more marked rise in blood triglyceride levels if it's eaten early in the night rather than in the morning. These mechanisms may explain the increased risk among night workers of developing diabetes and overly high levels of cholesterol and triglycerides. This is not surprising, since night workers eat and sleep at irregular and unconventional times, and often consume meals higher in sugar and fat than those of day workers.

In addition to affecting energy needs, sleep, and lack of sleep, have an important influence on appetite regulation (Figure 26). Two hormones essential for regulating appetite, leptin and ghrelin, fluctuate over the course of a day (Figure 27). This daily fluctuation is mainly the result of the alternation of periods of sleeping and waking. At night, leptin levels rise, telling the body it doesn't need to eat, and this signal is reinforced by the daily rhythm of ghrelin. Although ghrelin levels are elevated in the middle of the night, they decline at the end of the night, despite the organism's lack of food. The diurnal rhythm of these two hormones therefore means that during the night the body is not hungry, unless of course it has not had enough food the day before.

SLEEP RESTRICTION AND METABOLIC DISORDERS

Total sleep deprivation disrupts the nightly secretion of leptin. Levels of leptin, the satiety hormone, are thus reduced. Spending a sleepless night therefore stimulates the appetite.... Chronic sleep restriction also affects the levels of several hormones, as well as sugar metabolism. Regularly missing out on several hours of sleep changes the organism's response to carbohydrate intake in the morning. Thus, blood sugar and insulin levels are higher after morning muffins

BRAIN SCAN (MRI) SHOWING THE EFFECT OF A SLEEPLESS NIGHT

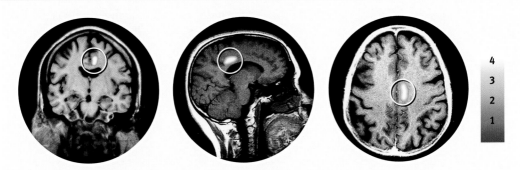

The right anterior cingulate cortex region is activated and the subject will crave food more if he or she can't sleep. The intensity of the activation in this region will range from red (1) to white (4) on the scale shown.

FIGURE 26   Adapted from Benedict et al., 2012.

if we have only slept for four hours that night, a sign of an abnormal tolerance to sugar intake, which is a risk factor for developing diabetes. This phenomenon may also be intensified by an increase in cortisol levels, cortisol being a stress-related hormone that responds to chronic sleep restriction. Cortisol interferes with the action of insulin and further disrupts sugar metabolism.

Sleep restriction is common in modern society. It particularly affects patients with sleep disorders and may contribute to an increased risk of metabolic disorders with advancing age. Sleep restriction causes a drop in leptin secretion and an increase in ghrelin secretion. These two hormonal changes cause patients to eat at night when they can't sleep. Regularly missing out on even just two hours of sleep a night would be enough to increase appetite in individuals who are already overweight! This can be a particular problem for obese patients with sleep apnea, who are trying to lose weight in the hope of better managing their sleep disorder (Chapter 8).

EFFECT OF SLEEP RESTRICTION ON THE SECRETION OF THE SATIETY HORMONE LEPTIN

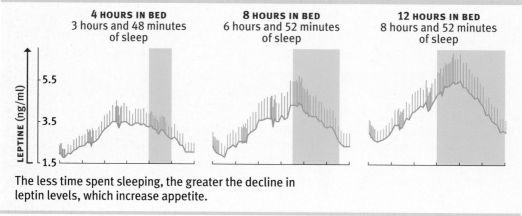

The less time spent sleeping, the greater the decline in leptin levels, which increase appetite.

FIGURE 27

Adapted from Van Cauter et al., 2008.

What Should You Take Away From This Chapter?

- The autonomic nervous system's more vegetative mechanisms predominate during sleep, especially during slow wave sleep.

- During REM sleep, the brain is almost as active as when it's awake, but the most active regions are not the same as those that are active during waking periods.

- Heart rate and blood pressure decrease during sleep and reach their lowest point during slow wave sleep. They rise again during REM sleep and after we get up in the morning. Sleep thus has a protective effect on the cardiovascular system.

- Sleep is a state of energy conservation. Body temperature and metabolism decrease during sleep.

- The feeling of hunger decreases during the night and sugar and fat metabolism slow down.

- Eating large meals late in the evening or, even worse, in the middle of the night can cause an increase in blood levels of sugar and fats.

- Sleep deprivation, even a few hours a night, disrupts appetite and metabolism and can also contribute to weight gain.

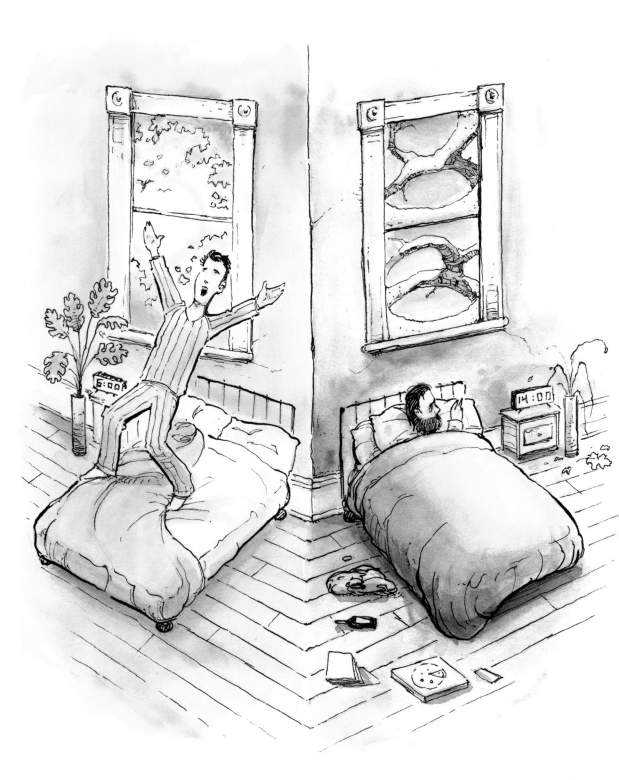

He found himself wanting when the north wind came.

CHAPTER 6

Waiting for Prince Charming

Sleeping, Waking, Light, and Mood

Sleep disturbances and fatigue are common features of psychological and psychiatric disorders. They can even worsen the distress that patients feel and increase the likelihood of relapse. Patients suffering from disorders like depression, bipolar disease, anxiety, premenstrual dysphoric disorder, or schizophrenia often have a chronically and severely disrupted sleep-wake cycle. Most of the medications used in psychiatry affect one aspect of sleep or another, or of circadian rhythms. Understanding the relationship between sleep disorders, the biological clock and mental health is therefore important. This knowledge has made it possible to develop treatment approaches based on controlling sleep-wake and light-dark cycles. Such approaches include light therapy, wake therapy, modifying the sleep schedule and social rhythm therapy.

THE BIOLOGICAL CLOCK INFLUENCES MOOD

A sophisticated time-isolation study of healthy participants (Boivin et al., 1997) showed that people's moods vary during the day, reaching a low at the end of the night and a peak at the end of the evening. This variation is partially explained by our biological clock's internal time and partially by our sleep schedule. During this study, participants lived in a private dimly lit bedroom on a twenty-eight hour schedule. The instruction was that they were to go to bed four hours later each day. This created a state of internal jet lag in which the effect of time zones on mood, vigilance and sleep could be studied. The participants recorded their moods on a scale ranging from very happy to very sad several times an hour for nearly a month. The study showed that slight changes in sleep schedule can affect mood, even in people who have no personal or family history of depression or psychiatric disorder. Actually, it's somewhat like what happens on Monday morning, when we go back to work after a very busy weekend.

It is in fact common, especially among young adults, to go out late in the evenings and lie around in bed on days off. These changes in sleep schedule are sufficient to shift our biological clock slightly to a later time of day. On Sunday night, therefore, it may seem harder to get to sleep. And Monday morning, when the alarm goes off, we wake up at the internal biological time when our mood levels are at their lowest. This is known as "Monday morning jet lag." If we feel less like working on Monday mornings, it's in part due to our biological clock! For those who recognize themselves in this description and who are seriously bothered by it, the best advice is to avoid changing bedtimes and wake times as much as possible. There's nothing wrong with a regular routine!

THE EFFECT OF LIGHT ON MOOD

Epidemiological studies have shown that people's moods and behaviour vary with the seasons in countries with pronounced changes in light levels. During the winter months, people often tend to sleep more, eat more carbohydrates — so-called comfort food — and experience a drop in energy and mood swings. The significance of these changes varies from one person to another along a continuum — at one end are individuals who are resistant and at the other, patients with severe disorders. Some people are therefore just as

energetic in winter as in summer, while others suffer terribly from changes in the seasons and can become depressed even after the autumn time change. This is called winter depression. A less serious kind of depression that does not meet all the criteria for major depression is called subclinical depression. People's genetic baggage seems to influence their vulnerability to seasonal depression. For example, it's interesting to note that Canadians of Icelandic origin are more resistant to seasonal depression than the Canadian population as a whole (Magnusson et al., 1993). This observation suggests that a process of natural selection may have occurred in Iceland, a country with very dramatic variations in seasonal light levels. As a result, people who were more resistant would have had an advantage in terms of survival and their ability to reproduce. The seriousness of other psychiatric disorders also varies according to the season. Patients with bipolar affective disorder, for example, have a heightened risk of relapsing into a hypomanic or manic phase in spring and summer, and an increased risk of depression in fall and winter.

WHEN SEASONAL DEPRESSION STRIKES

The expression "seasonal affective disorder" (SAD) was proposed in 1984 by Rosenthal and his colleagues to describe a recurring and seasonal-related mood disorder. The most common type is called winter depression. Sufferers fall into a major depression that begins in the fall, continues through the winter, and disappears in the spring and summer. These episodes recur, with spontaneous relapse and cure the following autumn and spring, respectively. The symptoms experienced by these patients are considered atypical, as they differ from those usually experienced during a major depression. Patients have a tendency to sleep longer at night, often complain of fatigue and drowsiness during the day, as well as of an appreciable drop in their energy, and they have a powerful craving for carbohydrates, often putting on several kilos during the winter (Figure 29). A shorter photoperiod, the length of time they are exposed to light every day (Figure 28), and lower levels of light in the environment contribute to the onset of this mood disorder.

The treatment of choice for winter depression is light therapy. Recent studies actually suggest that bright light seems to make the neurotransmitters important for maintaining mood, including serotonin, work better (Aan het Rot et al., 2010). The role of melatonin secretion in seasonal affective disorder has also been considered. Melatonin, also called the hormone of darkness, is secreted at night by the pineal gland in all animal species. In human beings, melatonin secretion begins early in the evening, reaches its peak in the middle of the night and stops in the morning; it thus occurs while we are sleeping. Melatonin is actually the hormone that indicates to the organism the beginning and end of the period of darkness called the scotoperiod. When individuals are exposed to bright light for sixteen hours a day and to darkness for eight hours at night — simulating a summer photoperiod — they secrete melatonin for a shorter time. When they are exposed to bright light for ten hours a day and to darkness for fourteen hours at night — simulating a winter photoperiod — they secrete melatonin for a longer period.

These observations raise the possibility that the higher level of melatonin observed in patients with seasonal affective disorder contributes to their state of depression. Other researchers think, however, that it's the timing of melatonin secretion that's problematic. For example, in 2006, Alfred Lewy and his colleagues in Oregon put

SEASONAL VARIATION OF THE PHOTOPERIOD (LIGHT) AND THE SCOTOPERIOD (DARKNESS) IN MONTREAL

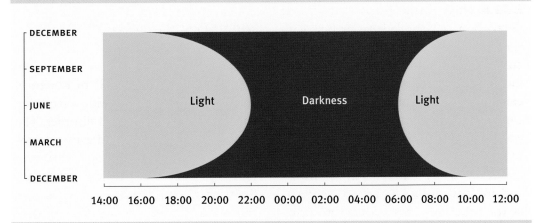

FIGURE 28

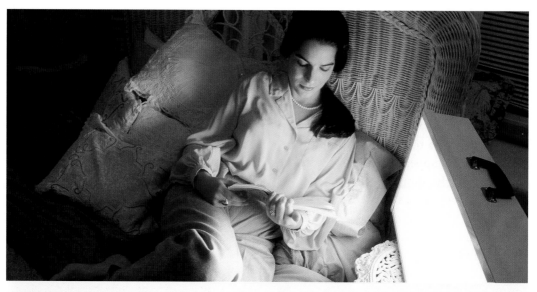

Light Therapy

Light therapy involves exposure to sources of bright light as a treatment for depression. Various types of lamps are marketed for medical use and are used mainly to treat seasonal affective disorder and circadian rhythm disorders. Light therapy is the treatment of choice for winter depression. Indeed, declining light levels in the natural environment when fall arrives is considered to be the main factor triggering winter depression. Light therapy trials have been done as part of the treatment of other mental disorders, such as major depression, bipolar affective disorder, and premenstrual dysphoric disorder. In the case of these illnesses, there have been fewer benefits than for seasonal affective disorder; in these cases, light therapy is therefore viewed as a complement to pharmacological treatment. The decision as to whether or not to use light therapy should however be made after discussion with a doctor, given the risks this approach involves. The most serious risk is that it might cause hypomania or mania in a patient with bipolar affective disorder. Other problems like headaches or irritability may also result.

To treat winter depression, light therapy sessions are usually scheduled in the morning and last from thirty to sixty minutes, but if it's inconvenient for a person to have these sessions in the morning, they will still be beneficial at other times of day. On the other hand, in the evening light therapy might be too stimulating and make it harder to fall asleep. During a light therapy session, it isn't necessary to stare at the lamp constantly. Patients are generally advised to set up the lamp about 30 to 60 centimetres away from them, for example on the breakfast table, and to look at it intermittently, as often as possible.

forward the hypothesis that these patients have a biological clock set too late in the day. According to these researchers, by administering light therapy treatments in the morning, this shift in the biological clock can be corrected, since exposing patients to light at that time shifts circadian rhythms to an earlier time of day. Light therapy appears to be slightly more effective in the morning than in the evening. This hypothesis is still being debated, as light therapy in the evening is also effective, although it does tend to delay biological rhythms even more.

Seasonal affective disorder also appears to respond favorably to sleep deprivation. Improved mood was observed in 52 percent of patients, compared with 29 percent of healthy subjects, after treatment using sleep deprivation. This rate of improvement is similar to that observed in cases of severe depression.

There is also a summer type of seasonal affective disorder. It's much less common than the winter type and therefore has been very little studied, making it still difficult to determine its causes. Excessive heat or other factors not yet understood, or even the lack of winter sports for those who enjoy them, may contribute to its onset.

GETTING INTO A GOOD MOOD

Sleep deprivation can have a negative effect on mood, even in healthy people. In depressed patients, on the other hand, manipulating sleep in this way often has an antidepressant effect. In the late 1970s, scientists observed that a good many depressed patients experienced mood fluctuations during the day. They often woke up in the morning in an obvious state of sadness that improved gradually as the day went on, until bedtime. This is called positive diurnal mood variation. This observation is the basis for the development of treatment trials that suggest to patients they stay awake one entire night. Therapeutic successes using this approach have been observed in 50 to 60 percent of depressed patients, especially among those with positive diurnal mood variation. Similar successes have been reported using total sleep deprivation (all night) or partial sleep deprivation (especially the last half of the night), and using selective REM sleep deprivation (the dream phases). These results are interesting as sleep deprivation offers a complementary approach to antidepressant use. Sleep deprivation, when it works, has an immediate antidepressant effect, whereas antidepressant medications usually take several weeks to work. We now use the more appealing expression "wake therapy" to designate this approach.

In clinical practice, however, this approach is rarely used, for several reasons. On the one hand, organizing suitable medical surveillance is difficult; on the other, the therapeutic effect varies from patient to patient and from night to night in the same patient. What's more, the antidepressant effect is limited in time and depression relapses have been reported after even just a fifteen-minute nap following a complete night of sleep deprivation. Deprivation may also cause a state of mania or hypomania in a bipolar patient. This treatment must therefore be discussed with the doctor. Studies of brain imaging have led to the discovery of a sub-group of depressed patients who

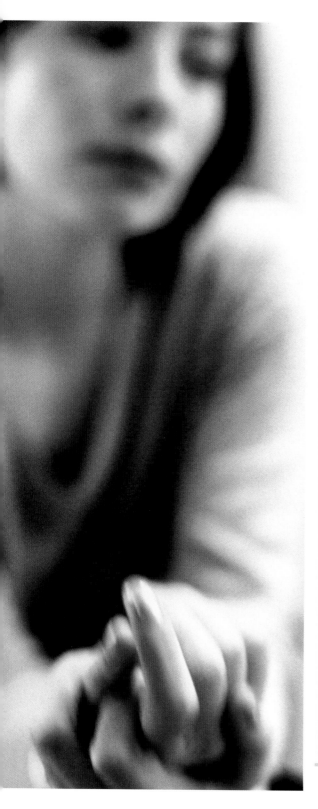

SYMPTOMS OF SEASONAL DEPRESSION

General Criteria

- Symptoms of severe depression develop at a particular time of year. In the winter form, symptoms of depression appear in the fall and continue through the winter. The summer form is much less common.

- Symptoms of depression disappear suddenly and completely when the season ends. Thus symptoms of winter depression subside in the spring and do not occur in summer. They reappear in the following fall and winter.

- This pattern of seasonal mood variation occurs for at least two consecutive years.

- From one season to another, social interactions, the length of sleep episodes, mood, appetite, weight, and energy levels change dramatically.

Symptoms of Depression

- Depressed mood, feeling of helplessness, feeling of worthlessness.

- Considerable fatigue, lack of energy.

- Tendency to sleep longer and difficulty getting up in the morning.

- Tendency to eat more fat- and carbohydrate-rich food.

- Weight gain.

FIGURE 29   Adapted from Rosenthal et al., 1984, and Lam and Levitt, 1999.

respond favorably to sleep deprivation and in whom brain activity is increased, as compared to the average person, in the regions of the brain responsible for controlling emotions, such as the ventral anterior cingulate cortex, the limbic system and the brain amygdala. In these people, sleep deprivation has the effect of reducing hyperactivity in these regions, returning them to normal functioning (Figure 30).

DEPRESSION AND SLEEP

Severe depression is one of the main causes of disability worldwide. Almost 12 percent of human beings are likely to suffer from it at some point during their lives. During a bout of acute depression, patients report feeling sad and depressed most of the time, for several consecutive weeks. Appetite is often negatively affected, sometimes causing substantial weight loss. Patients are often tired during the day, have no energy, and show a general lack of interest in their work, social activities, and life in general. They have disproportionate feelings of guilt, and it's not uncommon for these patients to think that death is desirable and sometimes to be quite open about their thoughts of and plans for committing suicide.

Almost all depressed patients report sleep disturbances, which in 80 to 90 percent of cases involve difficulty in getting to sleep, and sleep disrupted by repeated awakenings or cut short by early morning awakening. Conversely, some patients sleep more when they are depressed, a condition called hypersomnia. Hypersomnia is reported in 6 to

35 percent of cases, according to studies carried out to date. This change is often noted in the sleep of adolescents and patients with bipolar affective disorder and seasonal affective disorder. The internal organization of sleep is disrupted in these cases. There is a notable decrease in slow wave sleep during which a person normally recovers from the fatigue accumulated the preceding day. In a healthy person, the initial sleep cycles consist mainly of slow wave sleep, while cycles at the end of the night contain more REM sleep. Depressed patients may have much more REM sleep at the beginning of the night than healthy people.

SEEP DEPRIVATION AND THE BRAIN OF DEPRESSED PATIENTS

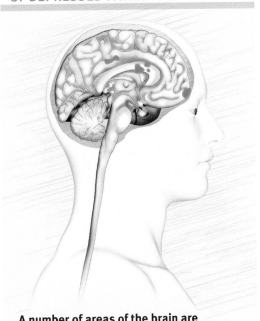

A number of areas of the brain are hyperactive in depressed patients.
These areas respond to sleep deprivation by decreasing their activity level, causing an antidepressant effect.

FIGURE 30   Adapted from Clark et al., 2006.

There is some evidence suggesting that circadian rhythms play a role in depression. For example, disruptions in circadian rhythms, such as a decrease in the amplitude of the body temperature curve and in the secretion of cortisol and melatonin, have been observed. Other studies indicate that depression can alter retinal sensitivity to light. Crossing time zones and working on atypical schedules (including night shifts) are risky activities for those with mental disorders.

The proportion of REM sleep is mainly influenced by the biological clock and is usually at its peak at the end of the night. Research on disruptions in the diurnal rhythm of REM sleep in depression led scientists at the National Institute of Mental Health, in the 1980s, to propose a model of depression based on a disruption in the biological clock (Wehr and Wirz-Justice, 1981). This model, known as the "internal coincidence" model, suggests that an internal discrepancy between their biological clock and their sleep schedule may contribute to the onset of depression in people at risk. This led to a treatment approach called "phase advance therapy," which requires that patients go to bed five or six hours earlier than usual. The approach seems to have beneficial effects in one out of two patients. The presumed role of circadian rhythms and the sleep-wake cycle in depression also serves as a scientific basis for developing new antidepressant medications. For example, agomelatine (not available in Canada) acts on both the melatonin and serotonin receptors and has an antidepressant action while also improving patients' sleep.

HYPNOGRAMS SHOWING THE STAGES OF SLEEP IN TWO MALES OF APPROXIMATELY THE SAME AGE, ONE BIPOLAR, THE OTHER HEALTHY

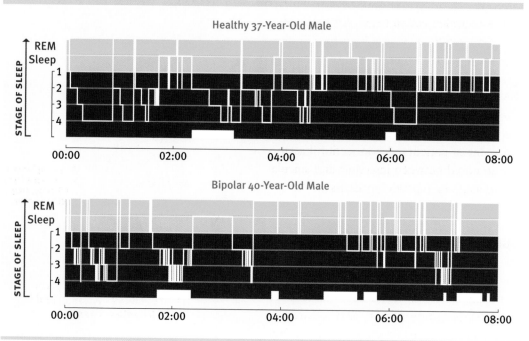

FIGURE 31

Hypnogrammes of two males, Dr. D.B. Boivin laboratory.

Other research will be needed to understand the circadian changes related to depression, but disruption of the circadian rhythms is definitely not the only factor involved, since changes in overall sleep requirements are also seen. A decline in the homeostatic need for sleep might therefore indicate that slow wave sleep is disrupted in cases of depression.

Women are approximately twice as likely as men to suffer from depression and insomnia. It's now clear that insomnia is a significant risk factor for the onset of depression. Nearly 40 percent of patients say they have experienced insomnia on its own (that is, without depression) in the years preceding the onset of the depression. This percentage is as high as 55 percent in patients with recurring depression (several episodes of severe depression). Meanwhile, roughly a third of patients report that insomnia started at the same time as their symptoms of depression. Another third report that insomnia started after their depression began. Insomnia that persists after a phase of depression also increases the likelihood of future relapses. In short, sleep disruptions, fatigue, and general lack of interest are the most commonly reported symptoms between depressive episodes and they occur in about 30 to 40 percent of patients. A connection has also been noted between insomnia and suicidal tendencies in depressed patients.

BIPOLAR AFFECTIVE DISORDER

In bipolar disorder, phases of depression and phases of mania or hypomania alternate in the same patient. Patients report that during their depressed periods they are sad and feel a drop in energy, a lack

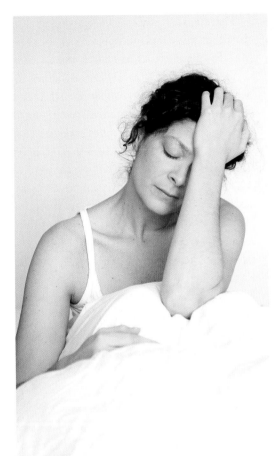

THE VICIOUS CIRCLE OF LACK OF SLEEP IN A BIPOLAR PATIENT

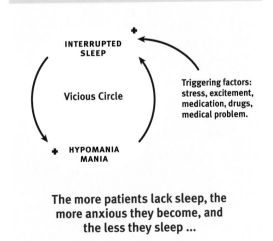

The more patients lack sleep, the more anxious they become, and the less they sleep …

FIGURE 32

109

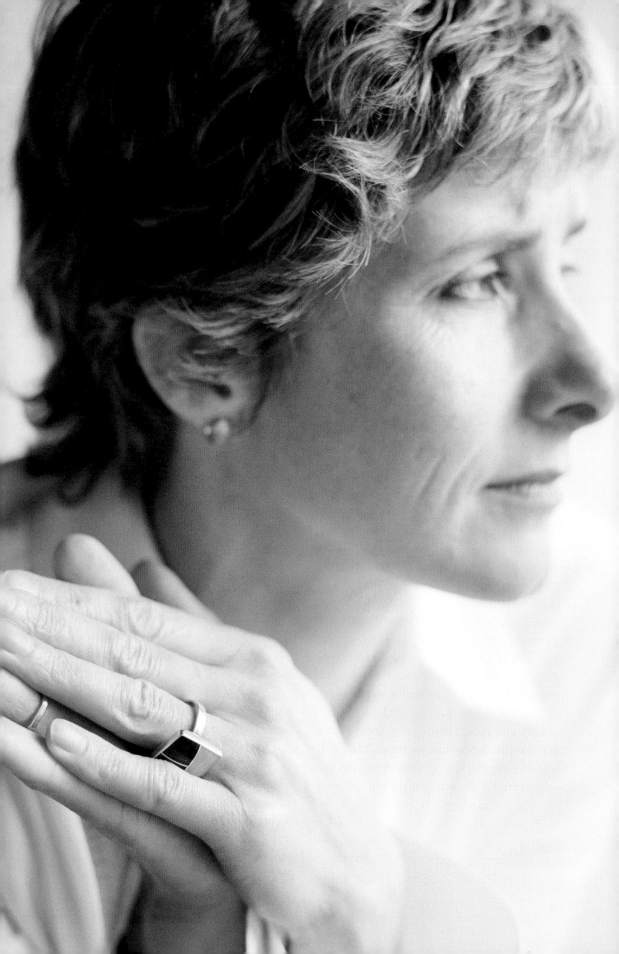

of motivation and general interest, often with recurring guilt feelings and suicidal thoughts. During these periods, they tend to sleep more and find it very hard to get out of bed in the morning, although some also say they suffer from insomnia.

In the hypomanic phase, patients have huge amounts of energy, a go-getting enthusiasm for several projects simultaneously, increased productivity and boundless libido. Alcohol and drug abuse is common. Sometimes these episodes are so extreme that delusions take over, resulting in loss of contact with reality. This is known as mania. Manic patients may become irritable, even violent, and disputes with the law sometimes occur. During these periods, patients may spend money extravagantly, causing financial and personal problems (for example, buying several cars, clothes, or very expensive audiovisual or computer equipment). During manic and hypomanic periods, patients generally say they sleep less, sometimes hardly at all, without feeling tired the following day. The phases of sadness and restlessness can last several weeks or several months each. On the other hand, some patients alternate rapidly between these phases, which last barely a few days and sometimes even a few hours in the same day. This is then called rapid cycling bipolar disorder, a state often combined with a strong feeling of anxiety, irritability and mood swings.

The causes of bipolar affective disorder are complex, but we now know that a genetic predisposition increases the likelihood of developing it. People whose parents suffered from it are therefore more at risk of developing the illness, especially when close family members are involved (father, mother, brother, sister). This disease stems from a malfunction in the neurotransmitter systems that control emotions.

Variations in sleep requirements are among the key factors that cause mood changes in bipolar patients. Changes in sleep organization may persist even during periods of remission (Figure 31). With experience, bipolar patients learn to pay attention to changes in their wake times and bedtimes. Thus, when they begin to sleep less and feel more energetic during the day, they recognize the onset of a hypomanic phase. They must then be especially careful and sometimes even see their doctor to avoid getting into a vicious circle where they may sleep less and less from one day to the next (Figure 32). This is a critical phase for them, since a lack of sleep increases the risk of mania. Sleeping regular hours in total darkness can help reduce the risk of manic decompensation.

Treatment for bipolar disorder is primarily pharmacological, as it's necessary to make up for deficiencies in the brain's neurotransmitter systems. In other words, the brain's chemical imbalances have to be corrected and mood-stabilized to avoid, in so far as possible, the cycling of phases of depression and hypomania and mania. As a result, patients often have to say goodbye to the state of euphoria and overflowing energy they feel in the hypomanic phase. Treatment trials using sleep deprivation and light therapy have been conducted in combination with medication. These clinical trials have been carried out in the depressive phase under medical surveillance, given the risk that hypomaniacal patients might suddenly become manic. Patients with bipolar affective disorder must not try these approaches on their own without having talked them over with their doctor. On the other hand, they may greatly benefit from trying an

PREMENSTRUAL DYSPHORIC DISORDER SYMPTOMS

General Criteria

- Symptoms of depression appear in the week before the period.
- These symptoms occur during at least five menstrual cycles in a year.
- The disorder is severe enough to interfere with work, studies, or social activities.

Symptoms of Depression

- Depressed mood, feeling of helplessness, feeling of worthlessness.
- Pronounced anxiety and mood swings.
- Anger and irritability causing interpersonal conflicts.
- Decreased interest in normal activities (work, school, social interactions).
- Difficulties concentrating.
- Lack of energy, lethargy, tendency to tire easily.
- Appetite changes, increased desire for certain foods (for example, "sugar cravings").
- Insomnia or hypersomnia.
- Physical ailments like headaches, weight gain, swelling and breast sensitivity, aching muscles and joints.

FIGURE 33

Adapted from DSM-IV (American Psychiatric Association, 1994).

approach called social rhythm therapy. Developed by Ellen Frank's team at the University of Pittsburgh, this approach aims to establish a schedule of daily activities, including wake times and bedtimes, mealtimes, and domestic and professional activities, as well as social activities. As part of a dynamic psychotherapy program and combined with the right medication, this approach has had better results than the conventional approach.

PREMENSTRUAL DYSPHORIC DISORDER

Between 3 and 8 percent of North American women experience severe mood disorders in the weeks before their menstrual periods. The symptoms usually start ten days before their period and disappear when their period is over (Figure 33). During this phase, patients feel extremely sad and experience a general loss of interest, anxiety, irritability, and sometimes even anger. They have mood swings that complicate their professional relationships and poison their personal lives. Sleep disorders are an integral part of these episodes. In fact, 70 percent of patients say they are getting poor quality non-restorative sleep, as well as feeling tired during the day. Some observations would seem to indicate that they need more sleep during this period.

The causes of premenstrual dysphoric disorder have not been clearly identified. Among the interesting findings that might explain the disorder is a deficiency in the circuits of neurotransmitters like serotonin. In these patients, a decrease in the secretion of progesterone and allopregnanolone (a metabolite of progesterone with beneficial effects on sleep and for fighting anxiety) has been noted. Insufficient melatonin secretion and perhaps a reduced sensitivity to its biological effect could also be involved. In severe cases, the use of anti-depressant drugs must be considered. Just as for other mental disorders, there has been some success with light therapy, but the condition must be studied further for this to be confirmed.

ANXIETY

Anxiety is the psychological disorder affecting the greatest number of individuals: nearly one person out of five will suffer from it during their lifetime. Anxiety is characterized by excessive worry about upsetting situations that might happen (Figure 34). Patients are thus overly worried about what unpleasant things might happen in the near or distant future. Their brain is constantly busy imagining possible scenarios and how to deal with them, scenarios that flood into their minds even at bedtime. In severe cases, uncontrollable panic attacks occur, often triggered by harmless incidents of the kind that do not endanger the person's life or safety. There is a very strong relationship between insomnia and chronic anxiety (Chapter 4).

SCHIZOPHRENIA

Schizophrenia is one of the most serious psychiatric illnesses. Its symptoms include cognitive impairment, the onset of delusions bearing no resemblance to reality, and hallucinations. The most common hallucinations are visual or auditory, with the patient seeing or hearing things that aren't there. But other kinds of hallucinations have also been described: having a bitter taste in the mouth, smelling revolting or rotting odours, feeling that someone or something is touching your body, watching your arms and legs move through space. Patients often develop delusions around their hallucinations. These symptoms generally undermine social relationships and frequently result in a patient feeling unusually suspicious and withdrawing from the world. Patients with schizophrenia often have disrupted sleep, with little slow wave sleep, and an abnormal, displaced sleep

CLINICAL SYMPTOMS OF GENERALIZED ANXIETY DISORDER

- Excessive worry with respect to upsetting events that might happen.

- Personal and social anxiety that is hard to control and incapacitating.

- Feeling of impatience, inner tension.

- Tendency to tire easily.

- Muscle tension.

- Memory loss.

- Irritability.

- Difficulty getting to sleep and nighttime awakenings.

- Restless, non-restorative sleep.

- Sudden panic attacks accompanied by rapid breathing, palpitations, dizziness, trembling, feeling of suffocation.

FIGURE 34   Adapted from the DSM-IV (American Psychiatric Association, 1994).

schedule. There are a number of reports of schizophrenic patients who completely reverse their sleep schedule, sleeping by day and staying up all night. This pattern, which definitely has a biological basis, makes their social withdrawal even worse.

Sleep disorders are an integral part of the clinical profile of all psychological and psychiatric disorders. Sleep disruptions increase the likelihood of developing mood disorders and relapsing into repeated episodes of depression. Several therapeutic approaches have been developed as a complement to conventional treatment with medications. Approaches like advancing the sleep schedule, wake therapy, light therapy and social rhythm therapy may be combined with pharmacological treatment to improve the management of mood disorders.

What Should You Take Away From This Chapter?

- In human beings, even those in perfect health, mood is influenced both by the biological clock and sleep deprivation.

- Sleep disturbance is a risk factor for the onset of major depression.

- Women are twice as likely to have insomnia and depression as men.

- Depressed patients often wake up feeling sad in the morning and their mood improves during the day.

- Seasonal affective disorder is a particular kind of mood disorder in which depression occurs in the fall and winter and goes away in the spring and fall.

- Decreased exposure to light is involved in winter depression. Light therapy is recommended to treat this condition.

- The importance of the sleep-wake cycle and circadian rhythms for mental health is at the heart of various treatment strategies that can be combined with pharmacological treatment of several psychiatric disorders.

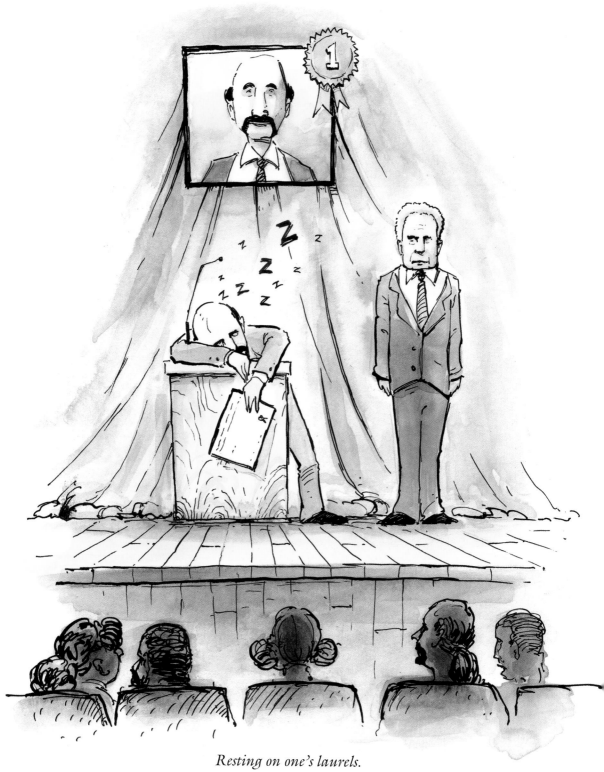

Resting on one's laurels.

CHAPTER 7

The Sleeping Beauty

Nodding Off When You Shouldn't

This chapter discusses wakefulness disorders known as disorders of excessive sleepiness. Excessive sleepiness is different from fatigue and stems from an inability to maintain appropriate levels of vigilance during the day. There are various medical causes for excessive daytime sleepiness. First and foremost are nocturnal respiratory disorders, especially sleep apnea syndrome. This is such a common problem in modern society that Chapter 8 is devoted entirely to it. Among the other common causes of hypersomnia is human narcolepsy, a debilitating neurological disorder characterized by irresistible urges to sleep during the day. Other kinds of pathological conditions such as idiopathic or episodic hypersomnia will be described. Disorders of excessive sleepiness require medical attention, given the potentially harmful consequences for patients and those around them. Lastly, various disorders of excessive sleepiness may be related to conditions that negatively affect the quality of nighttime sleep and circadian rhythms, or to the ingestion of sleep-inducing substances. An examination of lifestyle habits is essential, especially when patients are responsible for situations where the onset of sleepiness might be a risk to their health as well their safety and that of others.

NARCOLEPSY

Narcolepsy is a neurological disease classified as a wake-maintenance disorder and identified as a distinct entity in 1880 by Professor Gélineau. It's the second biggest cause of excessive daytime sleepiness after sleep apnea syndrome. The prevalence of narcolepsy in the general Caucasian population is between 0.02 and 0.18 percent. The

DO YOU HAVE
DAYTIME SLEEPINESS?

Take the following test to find out if you have a problem.

In normal conditions, how would you rate your likelihood of falling sleep in the following situations?

0 = NONE   1 = SLIGHT   2 = MODERATE   3 = HIGH

Reading while sitting down   ___

Watching TV   ___

Sitting, without doing anything,
in a public place   ___

As a passenger in a car for
an hour without a break   ___

Lying down to rest in the afternoon
when circumstances permit   ___

Sitting and talking to someone   ___

Sitting quietly after a lunch
without alcohol   ___

In a car, while stopped for
a few minutes in traffic   ___

SCORE ___

A score of 10 or more is a sign of moderate sleepiness while a score higher than 16 indicates severe sleepiness.

FIGURE 35   Adapted from Johns, 1991.

age at which symptoms appear ranges from five to sixty-three, with peak occurrence in adolescence and early adulthood. This is a crippling illness commonly involving four main symptoms — two considered major and two minor. Together these four symptoms make up what is called the narcoleptic tetrad. The major symptoms are excessive daytime sleepiness and cataplexy. The minor symptoms are bouts of sleep paralysis and hypnagogic hallucinations.

Narcoleptic daytime sleepiness is distinctive, as it involves a diurnal variation in vigilance, culminating in irresistible episodes of sleep (Dauvilliers et al., 2003). These irresistible episodes of sleep used to be called "sleep attacks," because of the irresistible need to sleep felt by patients. This kind of daytime sleepiness is different from that of sleep apnea syndrome. Furthermore, irresistible episodes of sleep occur not only in situations appropriate for sleeping, but also in unusual ones. The author recalls the rather astonishing case of a patient who slept while leaning against parking meters, even in the middle of winter! These sleep episodes result in relatively short involuntary naps (from five to twenty minutes) described as fully restorative. The level of vigilance then begins to decline again, resulting in another irresistible sleep episode a few hours later. These slow fluctuations in levels of vigilance during the day occur approximately every two to four hours: patients then feel an intense and recurring need for sleep that's hard to fight.

Patients who try to resist the irresistible need for sleep may enter an altered state of consciousness and experience dissociative and amnesic episodes called "automatic behaviours." These behaviours are indicative of a state that combines characteristics of both sleeping and waking. Patients can thus "wake up" somewhere without being able to remember how they got there, sometimes even having driven their car. Even though patients sleep in short episodes several times during the day, the total amount of sleep they get every day is essentially normal. Daytime sleepiness is by far the most incapacitating and treatment-resistant symptom of human narcolepsy. In the majority of cases, daytime sleepiness is the first sign of illness and persists into old age. Patients say they dream nearly 50 percent of the time during these short naps. In comparison, dreaming (or REM sleep) during daytime naps is quite a rare phenomenon in healthy people, unless they have been deprived of sleep.

Cataplexy is another major symptom of narcolepsy. It appears usually several years after the onset of excessive daytime sleepiness. Cataplexy is a key symptom, as it only appears in this condition. It involves temporary attacks of paralysis affecting the skeletal muscles — those attached to the skeleton, and necessary for maintaining posture — like those in the neck, jaw, arms, and legs. These attacks are usually partial, but they can sometimes be total, causing the patient to fall down, with a risk of injury. Cataplexy attacks are most often triggered by a sudden emotion like surprise, laughter, or anger. One example of a partial attack is the case of a patient whose head fell forward when she laughed or was telling a funny story, and who dropped her cup of coffee when she met a friend. There is also the example of a narcoleptic father who reported total cataplexy attacks, including falling down, whenever he had to lecture his son. The son understood that if he made his father

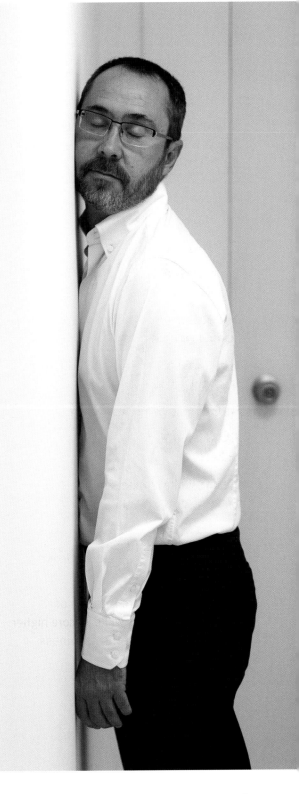

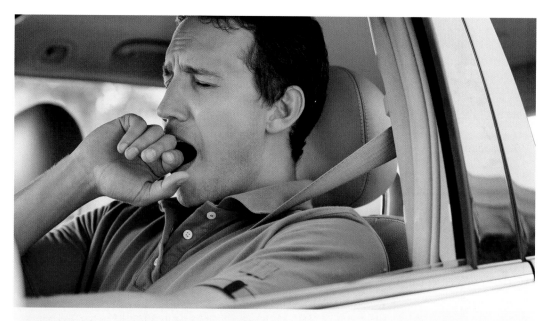

Fatigue or Daytime Sleepiness?

Fatigue is a subjective impression experienced as a state of physical or mental weakness. It's an integral part of the clinical profile of a great many medical conditions (Figure 36). In healthy people, fatigue is usually the result of a gradual loss of energy resulting from the accumulation of physical and mental tasks such as those related to work, sports, repeated stress, and even social activities. Fatigue may be temporary and acute or more insidious and chronic. Fatigue may also be the consequence of being awake too long or of a lack of sleep. In these cases, it comes close to what we call daytime sleepiness. Daytime sleepiness is the term used when staying awake becomes very difficult. For example, patients with daytime sleepiness will have trouble staying awake when they want to. Although in clinical practice we try to distinguish between fatigue and excessive daytime sleepiness, most of the time sleepy patients complain about fatigue and a lack of energy. The degree of sleepiness can be determined using a number of standardized questionnaires (Figure 35). Sleepiness can entail significant safety risks in work where constant vigilance is essential, such as when driving a road vehicle, maintaining heavy machinery, and handling dangerous objects (like butcher knives). It may lead to quality and productivity problems at work (for example, errors resulting from automatic behaviours when patients are fighting sleepiness), with sufferers going on disability, being fired or taking early retirement. Lastly, personal difficulties may arise, as family life and an active social life may be affected.

MEDICAL CONDITIONS CAUSING FATIGUE AND SLEEPINESS

Sleep disorder	Sleepiness
Periodic leg movements during sleep	Some patients have daytime sleepiness rather than insomnia. They feel sleepy when they get up and throughout the day.
Sleep apnea	Sleep apnea syndrome (especially the obstructive or mixed types) is usually associated with daytime sleepiness. The sleepiness persists throughout the day, becoming worse at the end of the day and during sedentary activities.
Narcolepsy	Irresistible episodes of daytime sleep, involuntary and fully restorative short naps.
Idiopathic hypersomnia	Long non-restorative naps. Excessive nighttime sleep.
Kleine-Levin Syndrome	Periodic hypersomnia.
Circadian rhythm disorders	Sleep schedule disorders with sleepiness at desired wake times. The sleepiness may cause difficulty in getting up in the morning or staying awake in the evening.

Psychological condition	
Major depression	Some patients — teenagers, for example — experience daytime sleepiness rather than insomnia.
Seasonal affective disorder	Hypersomnia, difficulty getting up in the morning, lack of energy, fatigue.
Bipolar affective disorder	Hypersomnia and fatigue in the depressed phase.

Medical condition	
Parkinson's disease	Daytime sleepiness often goes along with nighttime sleep disruption.
Hypothyroidism	Extreme fatigue.
Brain tumour, meningitis, encephalitis, and cardiovascular diseases	Sleepiness often associated with neurological damage.
Intoxication (alcohol, sedatives, narcotics)	Sleepiness and an altered state of consciousness.
Alzheimer-type dementia	Nighttime restlessness, disrupted schedule and sleep.

FIGURE 36

more impatient and emotional, the poor man would have a cataplectic attack, and his problem would be taken care of ... at least temporarily! Generally, cataplectic attacks are very brief, sometimes lasting from only a few seconds to a few minutes. This is why partial attacks are not always identified by a medical team. Furthermore, the seriousness of the cataplexy tends to diminish with age, and sometimes patients only have a few episodes in their entire lives. Even when patients have a total attack, including falling down, they don't lose consciousness unless the attack is accompanied by an involuntary nap, which occasionally happens and can be very disorienting. Cataplectic attacks are different from loss of consciousness and coma. They are also different from epileptic seizures since there is no loss of consciousness, urinary incontinence, biting of the tongue, and convulsions. Some epileptic seizures are nonetheless quite unusual and bizarre and it can also be hard to identify them (Chapter 9).

The other symptoms of narcolepsy are termed "minor," as they are less incapacitating and may be seen in healthy people who don't have narcolepsy, especially if they have built up a sleep debt. The minor symptoms of the narcoleptic tetrad are hypnagogic hallucinations and sleep paralysis. Cataplexy, sleep paralyses, and hypnagogic hallucinations are considered to be phenomena that have escaped from the phases of REM sleep. It's true that during REM sleep we are paralyzed and dream a good deal. However, the sleep paralysis normally observed in the phases of REM sleep can also occur in isolation when we are awake, in the form of attacks of cataplexy or sleep paralysis.

Occurring at the moment we fall asleep or when we wake up in the night, sleep paralysis is a temporary inability to move our arms and legs and open our eyes. It seldom lasts longer than ten minutes and ends by itself or in response to a slight touch.

The dream content or perceptual sensations sleepers experience during their dream phases can also occur on awakening. In these circumstances, people experience auditory, visual, or somesthetic (the feeling of being touched or that their arms and legs are moving) illusions, a little as if they were seeing, hearing or feeling their dreams ... but in a waking state. In this case, a person about to fall asleep or who wakes up in the middle of the night sees or feels things that do not exist. These are called hypnagogic hallucinations if they occur when falling asleep and hypnopompic hallucinations when they occur during spontaneous nocturnal awakenings.

Hypnagogic hallucinations can cause patients a great deal of anxiety, especially when they are accompanied by sleep paralysis or an intense or unpleasant dream. Unfortunately, this is often the case with narcoleptics. Explaining the mechanisms underlying these phenomena can reassure many patients. Familial types of sleep paralysis and hypnagogic hallucinations are reported without narcolepsy being involved. As in narcoleptic patients, these symptoms escaped from REM sleep can occur outside of REM sleep phases, like at bedtime, during the transition period between waking and sleeping, during nocturnal awakenings, or even during a daytime nap.

With age, the sleep of narcoleptic patients tends to deteriorate more quickly than that of healthy people. Nocturnal sleep

→ The contents of dreams or hallucinations can take very frightening shapes. Johann Heinrich Füssli, *The Nightmare* (1802).

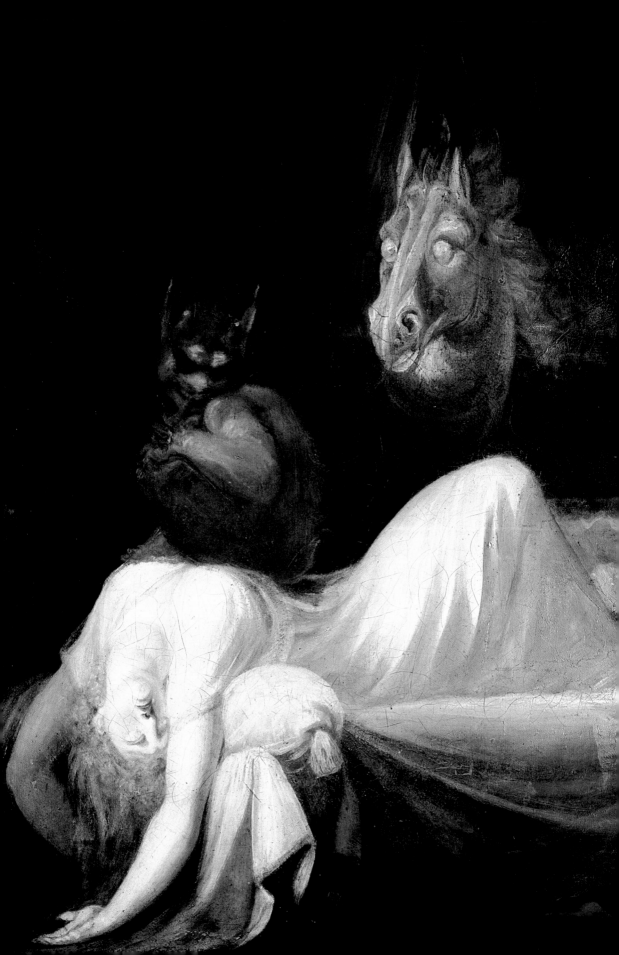

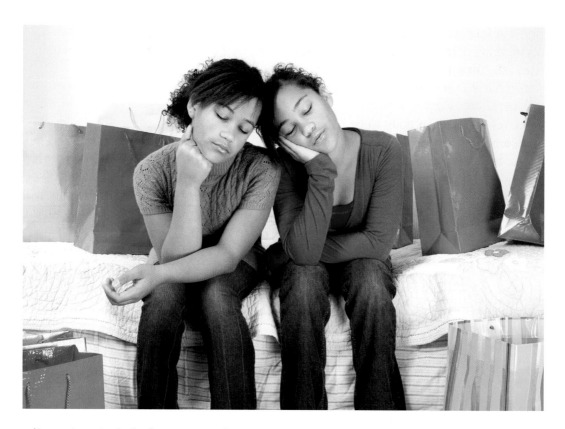

disruptions include frequent awakenings, less slow wave sleep, and a shorter period of time between falling asleep and the onset of the first phase of REM sleep. Their phases of REM sleep in particular are interrupted by many awakenings. The specific disruptions affecting the quality of REM sleep are a key factor in narcolepsy, and a correlation has been established between the deterioration of this stage of sleep and the onset of cataplexy. In addition, when pharmacological means are used to increase the consolidation of REM sleep phases (by administering gamma hydroxybutyrate of sodium, or GHB), there are fewer attacks of cataplexy. REM sleep fragmentation or the use of certain medications for cataplexy can sometimes cause what's called REM sleep behaviour disorder, a category of sleep disorders in which elements of waking and sleeping occur simultaneously. As they age, narcoleptic patients also have a higher risk of developing periodic leg movements during sleep.

A number of factors contribute to the development of this neurological disease. First, there is a genetic predisposition, as having a close family member with the disorder (father, mother, brother, sister) increases the risk of developing it. But other factors are also involved, as shown in the case of identical twins who share exactly the same genes but not the disease (one twin has it and the other does not). Certain environmental factors appear to contribute to the onset of the disease in patients who are genetically likely to develop it. These environmental conditions are not precisely known but could be related to disruptions in the sleep schedule or to childhood infections resulting in a series of inflammatory auto-immune reactions. In this type of reaction, the organism has an inappropriate defence response and begins to attack the parts of itself it perceives as a foreign body to be resisted. An exceptional 95 percent correlation has in fact been discovered between a susceptibility gene, the *human leukocyte antigen* (HLA) DQB1*0602, and the occurrence of narcolepsy with cataplexy. This gene seems to be involved in an auto-immune reaction leading to the destruction of the orexin/hypocretin system, located in the lateral hypothalamus and important for maintaining wakefulness. In addition, it's possible to document a notable drop in the neurotransmitter hypocretin-1 in the cephalorachidian liquid of narcoleptic patients with cataplexy (Nishino et al., 2010). The orexin/hypocretin system is connected to the circadian pacemaker and is part of the key centres for maintaining wakefulness. It's interesting to note that the control exercised by the biological clock over the processes of waking and sleeping is disrupted in narcolepsy (Dantz et al., 1994).

Some narcoleptic patients show no signs of cataplectic attacks. In these patients, diagnosis is made on the basis of sleep laboratory tests. The mechanisms underlying a narcoleptic disorder without cataplexy are less understood than the standard illness. It's likely that other susceptibility genes for the disease are present even in patients with cataplexy.

Lastly, rare cases of narcolepsy are the result of damage to the centre of the brain, in the diencephalus or brain stem, where regions that play an important role in controlling waking and sleeping are located.

LUMBAR PUNCTURE

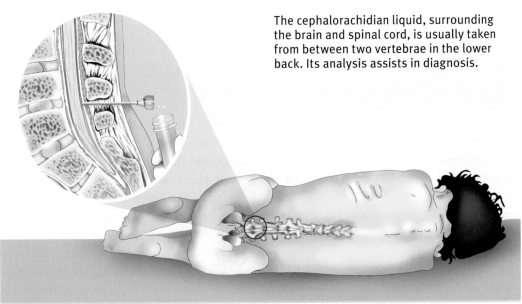

The cephalorachidian liquid, surrounding the brain and spinal cord, is usually taken from between two vertebrae in the lower back. Its analysis assists in diagnosis.

FIGURE 37

Narcolepsy is a disabling neurological disease requiring medical treatment. Medical history plays a part in its diagnosis, but screening in a sleep laboratory is especially important. The tests mainly involve making a polysomnographic recording of one or two nights of sleep and conducting tests of sleepiness during the day. The tests to measure sleepiness always include a "multiple sleep latency" test. During this test, patients lie down five or six times during the day in a dark, comfortable bedroom. They are instructed to go to sleep as quickly as possible and given twenty minutes to do so. Healthy people seldom fall asleep during all of these naps. However, narcoleptic patients generally fall asleep very quickly, in less than five minutes. Furthermore, episodes of REM sleep occur in at least two of these naps,

something that is much less common in healthy people. This observation indicates a disruption in REM sleep control in narcoleptic patients. The doctor may also suggest doing a lumbar puncture to check for a decrease in the levels of the neuropeptide hypocretin-1 (Figure 37).

The treatment for narcolepsy is symptomatic, that is, it consists of controlling the symptoms. There is no cure for the disease — you learn to live with it. The treatments are above all pharmacological and include taking medications that reduce daytime sleepiness and others that control the cataplexy. The anti-sleepiness medications are psychostimulants, products that promote wakefulness, such as modafinil (Alertec), amphetamines (Dexedrine) or methylphenidate (Ritalin). Psychostimulants work by increasing the transmission of monoamines in the central nervous system which are systems of neurotransmitters involved in wakefulness. These neurotransmitters are dopamine, adrenalin, and noradrenalin (Figure 38). The prescription of psychostimulants is controlled, given the risk of physical and psychological dependency.

A range of medications may be prescribed to decrease cataplexy, including taking GHB at bedtime, medications taken in the morning like those that enhance serotonin transmission (fluoxetine or Prozac), or noradrenaline (venlafaxine or Effexor). GHB seems to have a beneficial effect on cataplexy, perhaps because it helps correct disruptions in REM sleep during the night. Over time, GHB also has a therapeutic effect on daytime sleepiness, which means that some patients can stop taking psychostimulants. It isn't advisable, however, to stop taking

MECHANISM OF ACTION OF AMPHETAMINES ON THE DOPAMINERGIC NEURONS

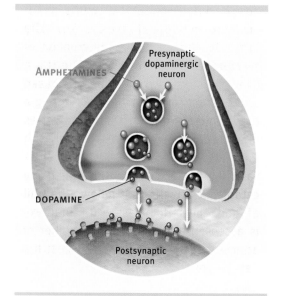

FIGURE 38   The effects on adrenergic neurons are not shown.

anticataplectic medications suddenly without a medical recommendation; their sudden withdrawal could cause a noticeable increase in the severity of cataplectic attacks and even result in prolonged seizures, a condition called *status cataplecticus.* Some medications marketed for other reasons (for example, fluoxetine, which fights depression) can also be used to treat cataplexy (and not depression, in this example). Other targeted treatments will be considered if other disorders are seen that disrupt the patient's sleep and condition even more (for example, periodic leg movements during sleep). Research is actively underway to discover new avenues of pharmacological treatment for narcolepsy.

In addition to using medications to control daytime sleepiness, cataplexy, and other related symptoms, reviewing patients' lifestyle habits and sleep hygiene is useful. It may be helpful for these patients to plan short frequent naps during the day so as to ward off uncontrollable sleep attacks in inappropriate circumstances. Driving a vehicle is an extremely important issue that must be clinically handled, given the public safety risks involved. It's not uncommon for patients to become depressed about their debilitating state. Depression will then require appropriate antidepressant treatment.

IDIOPATHIC HYPERSOMNIA

Some patients have an excessive tendency to sleep occurring both at night, during their main sleep episode, and by day, in the form of excessive daytime sleepiness. Research into the causes underlying this condition often yields no answers in a

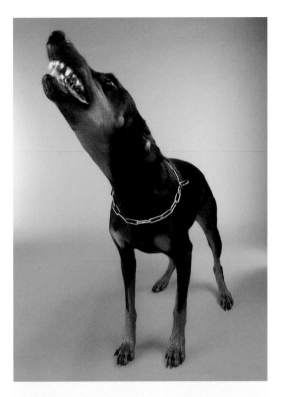

Canine Cataplexy

Spontaneously narcoleptic animals really do exist! Interbreeding narcoleptic Doberman Pinscher dogs at Stanford University in the late 1970s led to the creation of a colony of narcoleptic dogs. In dogs, a clinical diagnosis of narcolepsy is based on observed cataplectic attacks during a food provocation test. The test involves drawing a line in front of the animal, with dog food placed along it at regular intervals. The dog, excited by this, has many cataplectic attacks as it follows the trail of food. The seriousness of its cataplexy is assessed according to the number of attacks and the time taken to ingest the deposits of food.

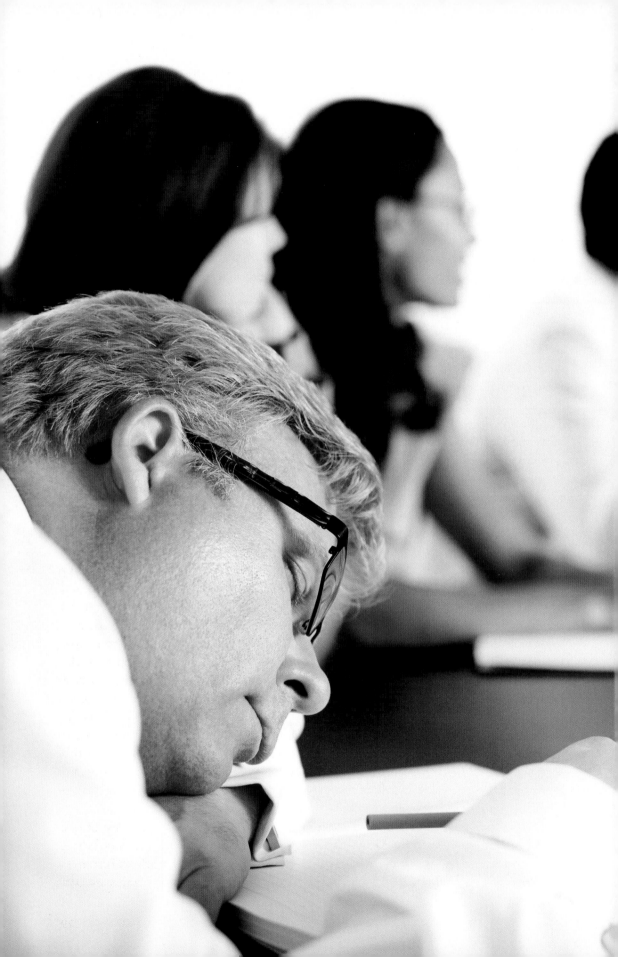

given patient. Thus, patients may have as much trouble staying awake as with narcolepsy, but without experiencing the other symptoms of the narcoleptic tetrad (especially cataplexy). Nor do they have other disorders that can disrupt their sleep at night or their vigilance during the day, like sleep apnea syndrome, periodic leg movements during sleep, or consumption of substances causing sleepiness. This condition is called idiopathic hypersomnia.

Idiopathic hypersomnia is less common than narcolepsy and develops during the second and third decades of life. Patients who have it tend to sleep too much at night, often more than ten hours in a row, and take long naps of an hour or more several times a day (Vernet and Arnulf, 2009). These naps are not, however, as refreshing as those observed in narcolepsy. When patients try to fight their sleepiness, they often display automatic behaviours they will feel embarrassed about later. Their sleep at night and during daytime naps includes more slow wave sleep than normal. This observation suggests an abnormally high need for sleep in these patients. As is the case with narcolepsy, treatment is symptomatic. It consists mainly of using psychostimulant medications to control excessive daytime sleepiness, and other medications may also be tried, since treatments are less effective than in cases of narcolepsy.

SECONDARY DAYTIME SLEEPINESS

Waking periods are part of the sleep-wake cycle. During this cycle, how alert we feel during the day is affected by how well we slept the night before. Conversely, activities carried out during the day can affect our ability to fall asleep and stay asleep the following night. Thus, any condition that disrupts sleep can interfere with its function of helping us recover from accumulated fatigue. Some patients with sleep disorders such as periodic leg movements during sleep (Chapter 9) or sleep apnea syndrome (Chapter 8) may suffer from excessive daytime sleepiness as a direct result. This is one of the reasons why a sleep laboratory investigation often involves a full night of recording; the goal is to detect these related disorders. It's also possible to organize mobile screening tests for sleep disorders, in other words, tests done at home. To do this, patients go to the sleep laboratory to have the equipment set up and get instructions on how to use it. They start the recording by themselves in their bedroom when they go to bed and return the equipment to the sleep lab the next day. The results are then taken from the equipment and analyzed by the medical team.

Sleepiness can also be a secondary effect of lack of sleep caused by patients' hectic lifestyles or the fact that they don't get all the sleep they need. Take the case of natural long sleepers, healthy people who naturally need more sleep than the average person. They might have a relative sleep debt compared with their needs and feel daytime sleepiness. In this case, increasing the number of hours of sleep at night fixes the problem, whereas this has no beneficial effect (and even possibly a harmful effect) on a patient with idiopathic hypersomnia.

Hypersomnia may also be caused by one of the circadian rhythm disorders, which disrupt the quality of both wakefulness and sleep. Fatigue and sleepiness are part of the clinical profile of several medical conditions (Figure 36). The underlying condition must therefore be treated and a symptomatic treatment for sleepiness also provided if it persists.

Finally, sleep disorders are very common in depression. Most of the time, they consist of difficulty in sleeping well at night, as well as daytime fatigue. Some patients, however, have hypersomnia instead of insomnia. This is an atypical, unusual kind of depression frequently seen in depressed teenagers, bipolar patients in the depressed phase and patients with seasonal affective disorder. In these patients, hypersomnia responds better to antidepressant medications than to psychostimulants.

PERIODIC HYPERSOMNIA

Kleine-Levin Syndrome is a rare and recurring cyclic hypersomnia disorder in which relatively long episodes of excessive sleep alternate with phases of normal or even exaggerated vigilance (Billiard et al., 2011). The phases of hypersomnia last from a few days to a few weeks. During these phases of increased sleep, a patient may sleep more than sixteen hours a day, become extremely hard to rouse, and display confusion and aggressiveness when forced to wake up. Other behavioural symptoms can appear: aggressiveness, excessive libido, hallucinations, and the impression of being disconnected from reality. It has even been suggested that this syndrome could be a type of bipolar affective disorder. Diagnosis is often difficult, as it requires being able to study the patient's case during the hypersomnia phases. Other kinds of periodic hypersomnia have been reported in women in relation to their menstrual cycles, especially during the week before their periods.

Several neurological disorders can cause severe sleepiness over the course of the day. People suffering from them have great difficulty staying awake all day and tend to fall asleep in sedentary positions, as well as in unexpected circumstances, at a restaurant with friends, for example, or behind the wheel of a car. For these patients, whose diagnosis and treatment require a medical consultation and regular follow-up, taking psychostimulant medication is recommended.

What Should You Take
Away From This Chapter?

- Daytime sleepiness is not just a matter of fatigue: its symptoms include difficulty staying awake and involuntary napping.

- Several neurological conditions can cause daytime sleepiness, including narcolepsy, idiopathic hypersomnia, and periodic hypersomnias.

- Narcolepsy has two major symptoms, irresistible sleep episodes and cataplectic attacks.

- The minor symptoms of narcolepsy are sleep paralysis and hallucinations. These symptoms can occur in healthy people.

- The sleepiness of narcoleptic patients is special in that it causes involuntary and irresistible naps that are short and totally refreshing.

- Sleep-inducing neurological disorders are treated by controlling their symptoms with psychostimulants.

- Planning regular short naps during the day can complement the pharmacological treatment of hypersomnia disorders.

- The sleep disorders that interfere with its restorative function can also cause daytime sleepiness disorder. These disorders require specific treatment.

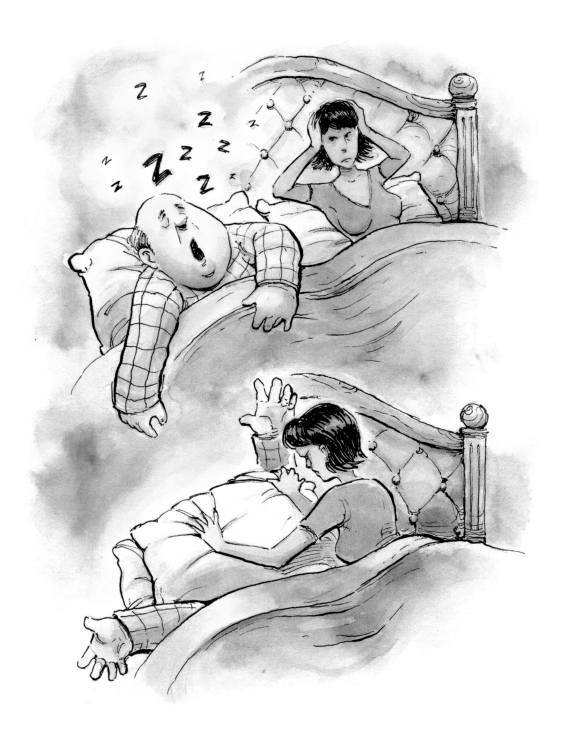

Sleep apnea can snuff out wedded bliss.

CHAPTER 8

An Unexpected Climb Up Mount Everest

Sleep Apneas

The workings of the human body undergo significant changes during the night. For example, breathing varies during the twenty-four hour day, mainly because the mechanisms that control breathing operate differently depending on whether we are awake or asleep. Going from a waking to a sleeping state is always accompanied by a gradual decrease in conscious control of vital functions. As a result, breathing control becomes more passive, weakening the stability of the response to the exchange of gases in the body. Several characteristics specific to the sleeper can greatly affect the quality of respiratory exchanges during sleep, in particular anatomical factors, related to the physiognomy of the head and neck, and neurological factors, related to the quality of respiratory control. These factors can be significant enough to cause periodic interruptions in breathing, called sleep apnea, or a marked reduction in the volume of air breathed, known as sleep hypopnea. These respiratory disruptions recur during the night and can be so frequent and prolonged that they greatly affect how refreshed we feel the next day. There's an interesting comparison to be made between the respiratory disorders and sleep these patients experience and those of mountain climbers who ascend rapidly to high altitudes — hence the title of this chapter.

Breathing disruptions during sleep can cause insomnia and excessive daytime sleepiness. They can also be accompanied by a significant drop in blood oxygen levels, with potentially serious consequences for the sleeper's cardiovascular health and brain function. Nighttime breathing disorders can thus be related to pronounced disruptions in cognitive abilities during the subsequent waking period.

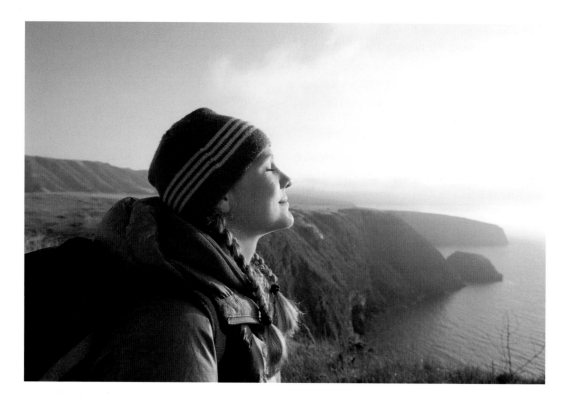

In less dramatic cases, efforts to breathe may encounter increased resistance to the passage of air through the respiratory system. This condition does not always cause breathing to stop completely or blood oxygen levels to drop. On the other hand, these respiratory efforts can also affect sleep quality to the point of disrupting the sleeper's functioning during the day. Nighttime respiratory disorders are a common problem in modern society; luckily, they can be treated relatively successfully. In this chapter, you will learn to recognize the signs, become familiar with various strategies for reaching a diagnosis and treating these disorders, and see what advice on sleep hygiene is given to patients who breathe poorly during sleep.

THE CONTROL OF RESPIRATION

Everyone knows that to survive we have to breathe, and we have to breathe air that's clean and rich in oxygen. But why is this so? Human beings, like all animals, produce organic waste from the energy burned in various cellular activities. Simply being alive and staying alive requires energy to be spent and produces biological waste in every cell in the body. We can simplify this by saying that every cell that burns energy also breathes and produces carbon gas, also called carbon dioxide or CO_2 (Figure 39). The carbon dioxide produced by cells throughout the body accumulates in small capillaries that irrigate the tissues of the various organs. These capillaries flow into progressively larger vessels called veins (Figure 40). Venous blood then flows to the right side of the heart to be pumped to the lungs.

Via the lungs, carbon dioxide is expelled into the surrounding air and the blood is oxygenated with fresh air. Freshly oxygenated blood then flows back to the heart, this time on the left side. From the left side of the heart, it's pumped into the aorta and the large arterial vessels. It then flows into smaller and smaller arteries called arterioles, and finally into the tiny capillaries that again irrigate the tissues of the various organs. In this way, oxygen reaches cells throughout the body, where it can then be used by cells to do their work.

Respiration, therefore, is how we transport fresh oxygen to the cells in our body and get rid of the carbon dioxide resulting from cellular work. Since carbon dioxide and oxygen are gases, the primary role of respiration is to control the exchange of gases. Because of this, the respiratory functions are sensitive to the concentrations of carbon dioxide and oxygen in the blood. Respiration thus speeds up when the concentration of carbon dioxide in the blood increases and the concentration of oxygen decreases. Conversely, it slows down when there is more oxygen and less carbon dioxide in the blood. Respiration can be improved by breathing more deeply or more often. With each breath, new air is inhaled into the lungs through a system of tubules that allow air to reach the lungs, the larynx, the trachea, and the bronchial tree. In the course of a normal breath, approximately 500 millilitres, or the equivalent of two-thirds of a bottle of wine, are inhaled and exhaled. Only two-thirds of this volume is used for respiration, with the remainder staying in the tubular system. This third is lost in what is called the "dead space" of the respiratory system. This is why it's much more efficient to take long slow breaths than to breathe quickly and superficially.

CONTROL OF RESPIRATION BY CARBON DIOXIDE (CO_2) AND OXYGEN (O_2)

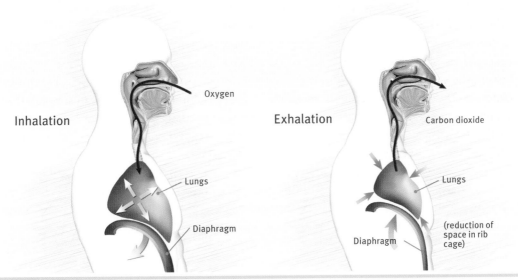

Inhalation

Oxygen

Lungs

Diaphragm

Exhalation

Carbon dioxide

Lungs

Diaphragm

(reduction of space in rib cage)

FIGURE 39

THE CARDIOVASCULAR SYSTEM AND ITS ARTERIAL AND VENOUS SUBSYSTEMS

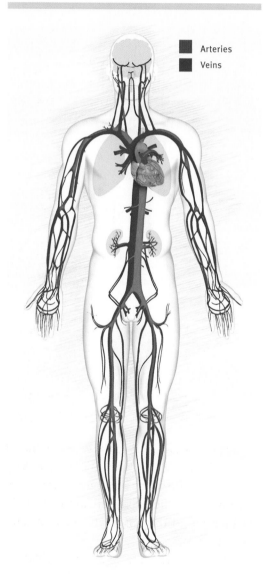

Arteries
Veins

The human body's vascular system is divided into two subsystems: venous and arterial. The venous system contains darker bluish blood carrying carbon dioxide. The arterial system contains lighter redder blood rich in oxygen.

FIGURE 40

RESPIRATION DURING THE SLEEP-WAKE CYCLE

During the day, when we are awake, we can change our breathing at will. We can therefore do relaxation exercises, consciously controlling our breathing, reducing its frequency, and increasing its volume. We can also choose to play a vigorous sport, which increases our energy and respiratory needs. We can deliberately choose to breathe through the nose or mouth. Generally, people breathe through the nose, hence the term nasal respiration. During some activities, like scuba diving, divers breathe through their mouths, since their nose is compressed by their diving mask. Air is breathed in through a tube attached to a tank containing oxygen (mixed with nitrogen). The upper part of the respiratory system is unusual in that it also has other functions. The mouth and nose are used for eating and smelling, the pharynx for swallowing, and the larynx makes it possible to speak. These common spaces are made up of a complex and sophisticated web of muscles, controlled by an array of cranial and cervical nerves. During childhood, we learn to use these muscles efficiently for speaking, chewing and swallowing without choking. Who doesn't remember their parents saying, "Don't talk with your mouth full or you might choke!" Several of these muscles are stimulated by the system that maintains wakefulness, giving them greater muscle tone during wakefulness to keep the pathways of the upper respiratory tract wide open.

During the transition from a waking to a sleeping state, the wakefulness stimulus to the oropharynx muscles is lost.

It's actually quite common for healthy people to experience a respiratory pause as they fall asleep. This decline in muscle tone increases as sleep becomes deeper. In several muscles of the oropharynx, particularly those with more than one function and that are therefore not restricted to breathing, muscle tone falls to its lowest level during REM sleep. Passive pressure changes in the oropharynx muscles, therefore, are what keep the airways open during sleep. Each inhalation creates suction inside the respiratory tube system. The soft parts of the system, located between the bones of the nose and the larynx, are sensitive to these pressure variations and may collapse periodically during sleep in some people. In addition, the shape of the neck and skull affects the geometry of the upper airways; these anatomical factors thus play a significant role in keeping the upper airways open during sleep.

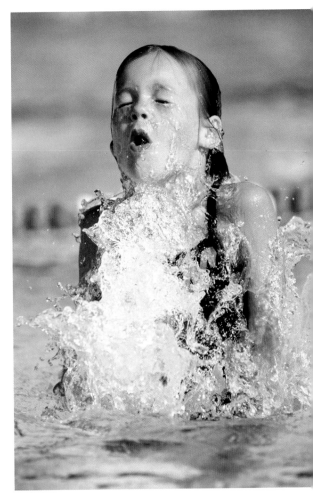

SLEEPING AT HIGH ALTITUDE

At elevations above sea level, there is a drop in barometric pressure. The air becomes thinner and less dense, resulting in a noticeable decrease in the pressure of its gases, especially oxygen. As a result, the air that gets into the lungs and the pulmonary alveoli contains less oxygen. This phenomenon becomes more acute the higher we climb above sea level. During a rapid ascent at high altitude, climbers get less oxygen with every breath, which lowers their blood oxygen level. The chemoreceptors sense this decrease in oxygen, and the body reacts by breathing more deeply and rapidly. In this so-called hyperventilation phase, carbon dioxide levels in the blood fall. The body reacts strongly to the drop in carbon dioxide by breathing more slowly. Thus begins the hypoventilation phase, in which blood oxygen levels decrease, and the cycle starts over again.

These cycles of respiratory oscillation between phases of hyperventilation and hypoventilation are typical of respiration during a rapid journey at high altitude. They are seen in waking periods but are more pronounced during sleep. Sometimes, the drop in carbon dioxide during sleep is so dramatic that it dips below the threshold to the point where the organism temporarily

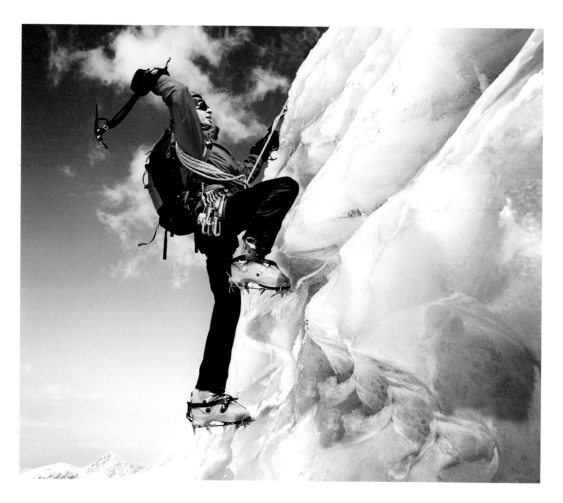

stops breathing, a condition called sleep apnea. Since all respiratory effort stops, this is called central sleep apnea.

During the first days at high altitude, sleep is interrupted by repeated awakenings and is not as deep as usual, with less slow wave sleep. Awakenings often occur at the end of a hypoventilation cycle and precede a hyperventilation phase. As a result climbers will complain about poorer quality sleep and often about fatigue or sleepiness during the day. A number of preventive treatments are available and have the effect of decreasing the reactivity of the respiratory response to the decline in carbon dioxide during hyperventilation phases. In the most

extreme situations, oxygen may have to be administered. Low-dose sleeping pills can enhance sleep quality without interfering with respiratory function. However, it's important first of all to be sure there is no underlying lung condition.

SNORING

Snoring is a noise associated with breathing that happens during sleep. It's produced by the vibration of soft tissues in the respiratory tree, between the nose and the larynx. As we have seen, muscle tone in the oropharynx slackens at the onset of sleep. This increases the likelihood that soft tissues at the back of the throat will vibrate. Lying on the back, in the dorsal decubitus position, causes the tongue to collapse toward the back of the mouth, making snoring even more likely. Any condition that increases air turbulence in the respiratory pathways can make snoring worse.

This is what happens in the case of nasal blockage (for example, during a cold), causing resistance to the passage of air, an increase in the suction effect in the oropharynx, or the tendency to breathe through the mouth. This is also why people who are overweight or obese are at greater risk of snoring than slender sleepers: in these patients, fat can be seen to have infiltrated the soft tissues of the oropharynx. A number of anatomical traits related to the shape of the neck and head can also be involved and explain why a tendency to snore may be more common in some families.

Owing to the anatomy of their respiratory pathways, approximately twice as many men as women snore, and the prevalence of symptoms varies greatly from study to study. One surprising fact is that during pregnancy nearly three out of ten women snore! Snoring and fatigue in pregnant women may indicate they suffer from sleep apnea. This apnea should be dealt with, as it can have harmful effects on the fetus (Komninos et al., 2011). Snoring is aggravated by conditions that further decrease muscle tone in the oropharynx during sleep. An example of this is when the sleeper has consumed alcohol or taken sleeping pills during the evening. Although occasional snoring is not dangerous for a sleeper's health, it can be a symptom of a more serious respiratory problem during

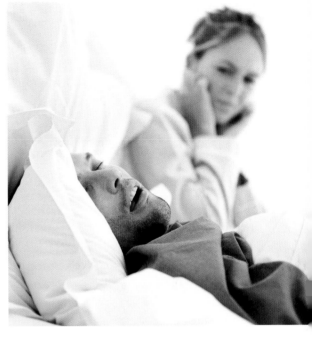

ADVICE TO REDUCE SNORING

- Lose weight.

- Limit alcohol consumption in the evening and abstain for at least two hours before going to bed.

- Avoid taking medications that cause evening sleepiness (including sleeping pills).

- Think about tricks to avoid sleeping on your back (for example, sewing a tennis ball into the back of your pyjamas).

- Consider taking a nasal decongestant when you have a cold or flu.

- Avoid sleep deprivation.

- Consider wearing a mechanical aid (for example, nasal dilators).

FIGURE 41

sleep, called obstructive sleep apnea. This syndrome, described later on, is deemed to exist when other symptoms that usually occur along with it are present, especially daytime sleepiness.

There are several methods that aim to reduce snoring (Figure 41). In general, a review of sleep hygiene is useful. Snorers are encouraged to avoid sleep deprivation because of "sleep rebound" — after sleep deprivation, an observed increased in length of sleeping time — and the increased risk of snoring that sleep rebound may cause. Not consuming alcohol for at least two hours before going to bed is recommended, as is always limiting consumption in the evening. Well-

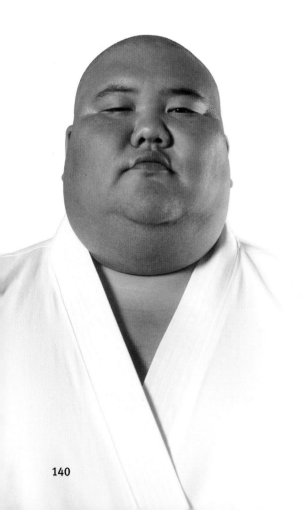

padded snorers are encouraged to lose some weight, especially by changing their eating habits and getting more physical activity (Schwartz et al., 2008). Recent studies have shown that controlling the sleeping position may also have beneficial effects in some apneic patients (Heinzer et al., 2012). Ways to prevent them from sleeping on their back should be tried, for example, sewing a tennis ball into the back of their pyjamas. This causes discomfort as soon as they roll onto their back and forces them to change position spontaneously during sleep. One patient with sleep apnea found it even more ingenious to use his wife's bra as a mechanical structure to keep tennis balls in place inside his pyjamas! Lastly, in the most serious cases of snoring, patients may consider wearing mechanical aids like nasal dilators. Surgical interventions are also possible. To the author's knowledge, there is no reliable test to predict which patients will respond favourably to these interventions.

SLEEP APNEA AND SLEEP HYPOPNEA SYNDROME

Some patients stop breathing periodically during their sleep. Apnea is when a patient completely stops breathing for at least ten seconds, and sleep apnea syndrome is diagnosed when this occurs at least five times an hour during sleep (Fleetham et al., 2007). Some patients stop breathing more than thirty times an hour! Breathing can sometimes be deeper and sometimes shallower, without stopping completely, however. Hypopnea is diagnosed when the decrease in respiratory volume meets certain established criteria. In general, the average number of apneas and hypopneas per hour of sleep will be considered in order to reach a diagnosis of sleep apnea and hypopnea syndrome. This number is called the sleep apnea and hypopnea index (AHI) and is used to determine how serious the syndrome is. The effect of these changes on the quality of breathing during sleep will also be taken into account in quantifying the blood oxygen saturation level. During the waking period, the blood oxygen saturation level hovers around 98 to 100 percent. In serious cases of sleep apnea, this saturation level can drop to as low as 55 to 60 percent, with harmful cardiovascular, metabolic and brain repercussions (Jean-Louis et al., 2008). Metabolic disorders that increase the risk of developing diabetes have in fact been seen in apneic patients. These metabolic disorders are a function of the seriousness of the medical condition (Bulcun et al., 2012).

The type of sleep apnea a patient has is also identified during screening recordings. There are two main kinds of apnea, central and obstructive. Central apnea occurs when there is no respiratory command (as described with regard to high-altitude climbers). In central apnea, there is no apparent effort to breathe and no volume of air goes through the lungs. Obstructive apnea is instead the result of an obstruction in the airway during breathing. During obstructive apnea, major efforts are made to breathe, but there is no air circulation in the respiratory pathways. Central sleep apnea syndrome affects approximately one out of ten apneic patients. Obstructive sleep apnea syndrome affects roughly nine out of ten apneic patients. That said, "pure" cases are very rare and most of the time a patient has both types of apnea, with either the central or obstructive type predominating (a mixed profile) (Figure 42).

TYPES OF SLEEP APNEA: CENTRAL APNEAS, OBSTRUCTIVE APNEAS, AND MIXED APNEAS

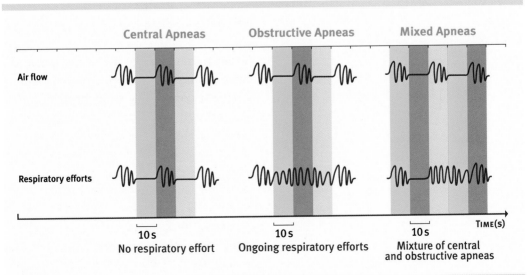

FIGURE 42

Obstructive sleep apnea syndrome is an increasingly common problem in modern society; the main explanation is an increase in the problems of overweight and obesity and more recent acknowledgement of the issue by the medical community. The typical clinical profile of a patient with this syndrome is that of an obese male, with a short thickset neck, who snores alarmingly during his sleep. However, it's important to keep an open mind, as this syndrome can also occur in slender patients whose only complaint is that they snore and are tired during the day. It can also occur in women, especially after menopause. Repeated attempts to breathe often end in a sudden awakening accompanied by an intense effort to clear the blockage, usually with a thundering noise. Some apneic patients snore so loudly that the noise of their snoring can exceed the environmental standards for nighttime noise. Snoring louder than 85 decibels has been reported (the noise level inside a car in urban traffic) in apneic patients. Getting the partner's side of the story is therefore very useful for the doctor. Bruises caused by the partner jabbing her elbow into the patient's ribs to get him to stop snoring speak for themselves.... It's not uncommon for a couple to sleep in separate bedrooms for this reason, but sleepers in neighbouring bedrooms may still complain about the patient's snoring.

Sleep apnea syndrome greatly disrupts the quality of nighttime sleep, interrupting it with frequent awakenings. The sleeper often gets up in the morning more tired than at bedtime and drags this fatigue around all day. This is in fact the most common cause of excessive daytime sleepiness. In sleep apnea syndrome, sleepiness persists all day, tends to get worse as the hours go by, and is not relieved by a nap. Patients may actually wake up even more tired after a nap, especially if it was interrupted by apneas.

Repeated awakenings during sleep and the decline in blood oxygen levels can contribute to the onset of daytime sleepiness and a range of cognitive disorders (Jean-Louis et al., 2012). Apneic patients may thus have concentration and memory difficulties and be less productive at work. They may have trouble remaining as vigilant as they should during their waking periods, increasing the risk of workplace and driving accidents. Patients must become aware of these risks and avoid situations that are potentially dangerous for their safety and that of others. People should never continue to drive when they feel very tired behind the wheel. When apneic patients try to fight their daytime sleepiness, automatic behaviours may take over, along with factual amnesia. If they are behind the wheel of their car, they may "wake up" in a particular place, often unknown to them, without remembering how they got there. Mood changes and irritability can occur, and untreated apneics often report libido problems and erectile dysfunction.

The periodic decline in blood oxygen levels puts significant stress on the cardiovascular system. As a result, cardiovascular disorders like the onset of high blood pressure or a heightened risk of coronary disease and heart attack in apneic patients have been noted, especially if their syndrome is severe.

Patients with obstructive apneas tend to experience more excessive daytime sleepiness, while those with the central type more often report difficulty sleeping soundly. On the other hand, nearly

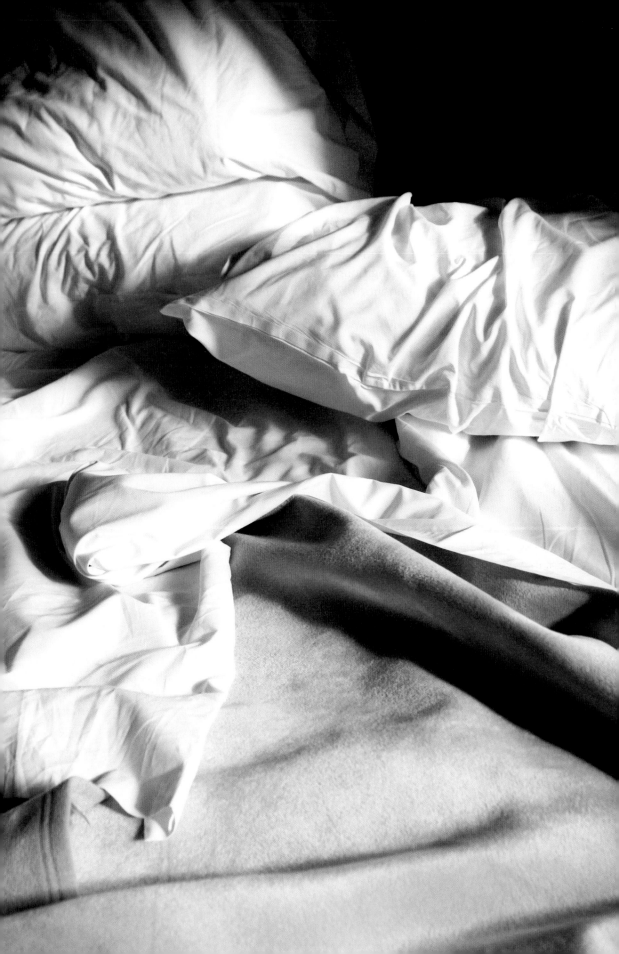

TREATING SLEEP APNEA WITH CONTINUOUS POSITIVE AIRWAY PRESSURE VENTILATION (CPAP)

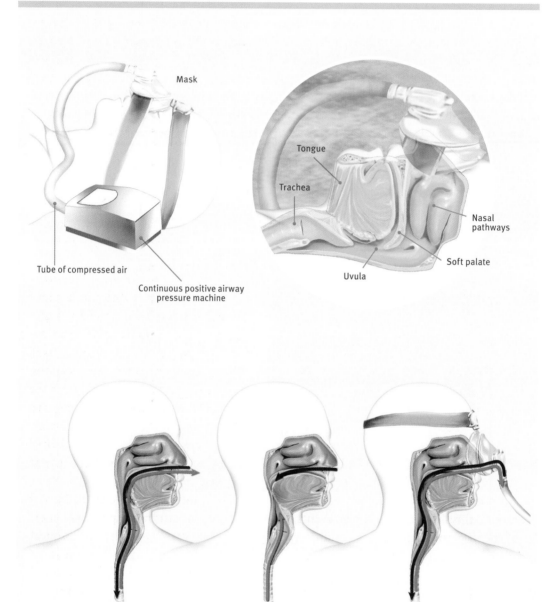

FIGURE 43

one out of two patients with obstructive apneas complains about restless sleep, and with age, patients tend to develop insomnia. The recurring awakenings typical of this type of syndrome can trigger sleepwalking episodes and even REM sleep behaviour disorder, two conditions in which the boundaries between states of vigilance are blurred (Chapter 9).

Various risk factors influencing the onset of a sleep apnea syndrome have been discovered. Obesity is a major risk factor; nearly one out of four obese patients suffers from it, with this risk climbing as waist circumference increases. As with snoring, familial factors linked to the anatomy of the head and neck are also involved. As we have already seen, there is a loss of oropharyngeal muscle tone during sleep. And when the airways are narrow, oropharyngeal muscle contractions are not enough to keep the airways open during sleep. One or more blockages then occur repeatedly in the upper respiratory pathways during sleep. Drinking alcohol or taking sleeping pills or any sleep-inducing substance can reduce muscle tone in the oropharynx even more during sleep. These products can also disrupt the respiratory system's response to the drop in blood oxygen levels and raise the arousal threshold during apneic events. All of these factors can make a condition already deemed problematic even worse.

Central apnea syndrome, meanwhile, is often associated with other medical conditions, such as heart failure, narcotic overdose, various severe neurological diseases, like those stemming from encephalitis, a stroke, a tumour, or poorly controlled diabetes. These diseases all affect one or another of the mechanisms controlling breathing during sleep.

The best treatment for obstructive and mixed sleep apnea syndrome is to use a Continuous Positive Airway Pressure machine or CPAP machine (Figure 43). This machine forces compressed air through the nose into the patient's respiratory pathways during the night. It's really an "air pump" to keep the airways open during sleep. A breaking-in period is needed so the air pressure can be adjusted. It's important for patients to have access to a technical support service for adjusting their machine. Medical follow-up is also necessary to assess their response to treatment. These conditions can have a major influence on patients' adherence to treatment and its success.

This treatment is strongly recommended in severe cases of sleep apnea and ideally the appliance is worn every night. Other therapeutic approaches may be proposed for very mild to moderate cases, including nighttime prostheses. Various kinds of equipment are on the market for this purpose. Some work by pulling the jaw forward, while others pull the tongue forward. These appliances fit much better and are more comfortable and effective if they are inserted by a dentist.

Finally, some patients prefer the idea of having their nocturnal respiratory blockage surgically corrected. The first surgical treatments developed for treating sleep apneas were highly invasive and involved performing a tracheotomy, or creating an opening into the trachea directly through the neck. Today, more sophisticated approaches are available, including uvulopalatopharyngoplasty. The purpose of this technique is to enlarge the oropharyngeal cavity by removing soft tissues like the uvula and the soft palate. However, blockages often form in many places and apneas can recur after surgery. Medical follow-up is thus required. Other extreme surgical approaches, called bariatric surgery, are used to treat morbid obesity. Their aim is to reduce food absorption in the gastrointestinal tract and in so doing promote dramatic weight loss.

Reviewing lifestyle habits and maintaining a healthy weight are important for apneic patients. Sometimes just losing weight is enough to treat mild cases of sleep apnea. Still, this approach on its own is often not enough and the use of oral prostheses or a continuous positive airway pressure appliance may be suggested. The advice given to reduce snoring should also be followed by apneic patients. They should avoid consuming alcohol, sleeping pills, and any respiratory depressant during the evening. They should also take steps to prevent sleeping on their back and avoid situations causing additional sleep deprivation as much as possible.

Breathing disruptions at night have serious consequences for sleepers' health, since the drop in blood oxygen levels is harmful for the heart, the brain and the entire organism. Apneic sleepers are often unaware of these respiratory interruptions. This disorder can be treated relatively successfully but requires medical supervision and proper follow-up. Talk to your doctor about it, if you snore loudly at night and suffer from excessive sleepiness. If this is the case, you should be especially careful in circumstances where a decrease in vigilance could have harmful consequences (when driving a vehicle or using dangerous equipment).

What Should You Take Away From This Chapter?

- The environment influences respiratory exchanges, which in turn affect sleep.

- Breathing control changes during sleep, when it may deteriorate.

- Anatomical factors related to the shape of the head and neck predispose some individuals to snoring and sleep apneas.

- Sleep apnea syndrome is characterized by repeated and prolonged inter-ruptions in breathing during sleep. In severe cases, oxygen levels in the blood drop dangerously.

- The decline in blood oxygen levels, repeated efforts to breathe and sleep disruptions related to sleep apneas pose a risk to cardiovascular health.

- Sleep apnea syndrome is the most common cause of excessive daytime sleepiness and must be considered in patients who snore loudly at night and sleep during the day.

- There are effective treatments to control sleep apneas, including wearing a continuous positive airway pressure appliance (CPAP).

- Apneic patients should make changes in their lifestyle habits and consider losing weight if they are too heavy.

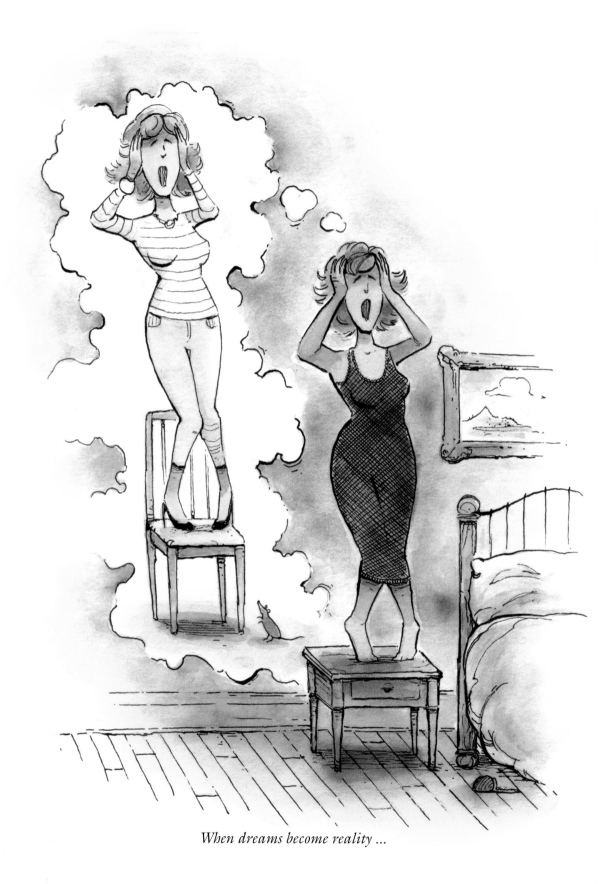

When dreams become reality ...

CHAPTER 9

Bedtime Stories

Nighttime Restlessness Disorders

This chapter looks at medical conditions that disrupt sleep and involve abnormal movements or behaviours during the night. One component of all the sleep disorders described in this chapter is nighttime restlessness. These disorders may belong to the category of parasomnias — states of motor restlessness during sleep, especially during the transitions between stages of sleep. Sleep myoclonus, sleepwalking, night terrors, and sleep-talking are some examples. Parasomnias are not necessarily considered abnormal, as is commonly noted when they occur during childhood. The seriousness of these phenomena, the age of onset and the repercussions for the quality of life of patients are some of the factors that determine whether these disorders require medical attention. Sometimes, however, nighttime restlessness is a sign of a neurological disorder that disrupts sleep, in particular the mechanisms governing muscle

control during sleep. The classic example is REM sleep behaviour disorder. Periodic leg movements during sleep are also described in this chapter, as they often cause patients to move their legs, get up and walk around at night to find relief. Lastly, bouts of nighttime restlessness can be signs of a neurological problem like epilepsy. These disorders are sometimes hard to evaluate and therefore require a medical consultation and in-depth studies in a sleep lab.

PARASOMNIAS

Parasomnias are sleep disorders characterized by motor restlessness and behaviours that often appear stereotyped and bizarre occurring during sleep. This fascinating class of phenomena provides evidence of a zone of ambivalence between normal sleeping and waking activities (Mahowald et al., 2011). Indeed, during episodes of parasomnia, patients are deeply asleep but behave as if they were awake. An episode of parasomnia can even be induced in susceptible patients by partially waking them up (sleepwalking, for example) while they are sleeping. There are two main classes of parasomnia: those that occur during REM sleep (the dream phases) and those occurring during the other phases of sleep — non-REM parasomnias. Sleepwalking and night terrors are examples of non-REM parasomnias that often occur during slow wave sleep and are also sometimes called slow-wave parasomnias. Since slow wave sleep is concentrated early in the night and REM sleep at the end of the night, non-REM and REM parasomnias are more common at the beginning and end of the night, respectively (Figure 45). Awakenings during stages of slow wave sleep are usually associated with temporary confusion. Thus, some degree of disorientation accompanies slow-wave parasomnias: patients vaguely remember the dream or nightmare they had just before waking up. In comparison, patients who wake up during an episode of REM-sleep parasomnia come to their senses faster and often tell a complicated story about their dream that corresponds to their inappropriate movements during the night. It often takes enormous effort to wake up a patient experiencing an episode of parasomnia, whether it occurs in slow wave sleep or REM sleep.

SLEEP MYOCLONUS

Sleep myoclonus involves sudden jerky movements during the transition between waking and sleeping and is caused by a sudden loss of muscle tone at the onset of sleep. No treatment is required, as this is a normal occurrence. Before going to bed, a period of relaxation to relieve daily stress might help lower muscle tension and cause myoclonus to occur less often.

SLEEP-TALKING

Some people talk during their sleep. This is called somniloquy, or sleep-talking, and often accompanies other kinds of parasomnia, such as sleepwalking or night terrors. Sleep-talking may occur during other stages of sleep in addition to slow wave sleep, and even in REM sleep. Sleep-talking requires neither medical investigation nor any special treatment (unless the patient reveals embarrassing secrets). Reviewing sleep hygiene, drinking less alcohol in the evening, and more regular bedtimes and wake-up times should always be considered, especially if the problem becomes frequent and disturbs the partner's sleep.

SLEEPWALKING

Sleepwalking, or somnambulism, involves episodes of nighttime restlessness during which those affected are sleeping deeply but behave in ways that seem as coordinated as if they were awake. Sleepers may behave in stereotypical ways using mechanical gestures. During episodes of sleepwalking, sleepers may wander around with no apparent purpose, eat, or do irrational things like urinate in the dryer or move objects they will then look for the

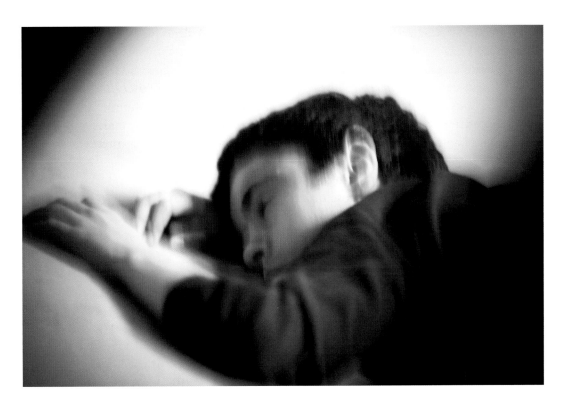

next day. In the most severe cases, sleep-walkers may put themselves in danger, by leaving their home in their pyjamas or injuring themselves accidentally by tripping over an obstacle, for example. Cases of people jumping out of a window or of violent or inappropriate sexual behaviour have also been reported. Attacks of sleep-walking occur during non-REM sleep, in particular during slow wave sleep. This means they are more common in the early hours of the night, when stage 3 and stage 4 sleep predominate.

This connection between sleepwalking and the stages of slow wave sleep explains why sleepwalkers are often hard to rouse and confused when they are forced to wake up. Confusion on awakening from sleep is a result of a phenomenon called sleep inertia. Since children have much more slow wave sleep than adults, they are more likely to have episodes of sleepwalking. Some studies report that nearly one in five children has experienced them. Sleepwalking and night terrors are actually so common during childhood that they are considered to be a normal part of brain growth and maturation. It's less common for sleepwalking to persist into adulthood, with approximately one in twenty-five people experiencing it. In these cases a genetic predisposition seems to be involved, and there are families in which several members are affected right through to old age. Underlying sleep disorders, such as a nocturnal respiratory disorder, must also be ruled out (Cao and Guilleminault, 2010).

Sleepwalking in children does not usually require any treatment. The best attitude for parents to take is to comfort their child and gently suggest they go

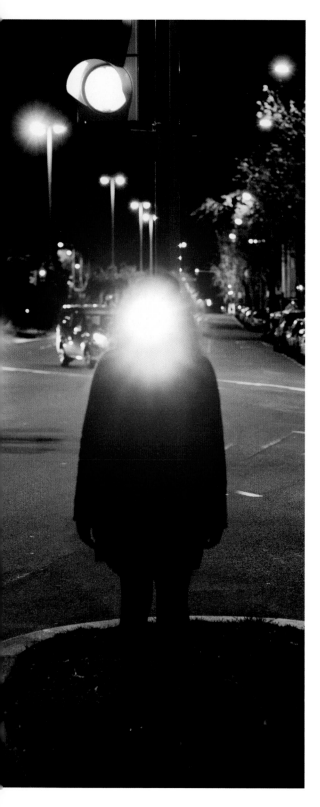

back to bed. Since the arousal threshold is higher during slow wave sleep, it can be quite difficult to wake up a sleepwalker, but you must not hesitate to do so if the person is in danger: about to jump off a balcony, for example, or do something reprehensible. In adults, it can sometimes be necessary to treat sleepwalking. First, sleep hygiene must be reviewed. Since episodes occur during slow wave sleep, patients must learn to avoid as much as possible situations like sleep deprivation that trigger more of these stages of sleep. Drinking alcohol in the evening, especially in large amounts, and taking some types of sleeping pills can make the problem worse. Their consumption must therefore be reviewed. Episodes of nocturnal behaviours involving amnesia and a dissociative state sometimes causing conflicts with the law are known to have occurred (Umanath et al., 2011). In most cases, these episodes are associated with a dysfunctional family environment or the excessive consumption of alcohol or sedatives in the evening. In severe cases, medication may be considered to reduce the number of sleepwalking episodes. Some of these products work by reducing the amount of slow wave sleep. These approaches must however be discussed with a doctor, and patients must avoid suddenly ceasing to take the recommended medication.

Sometimes sleepwalking is caused by other sleep disorders like sleep apnea, periodic leg movements during sleep, nocturnal epilepsy, or some medications used in psychiatry. These attacks can also occur during menstrual periods in some women. In short, various conditions often cause sleep disruptions that can trigger

Sleep Deprivation

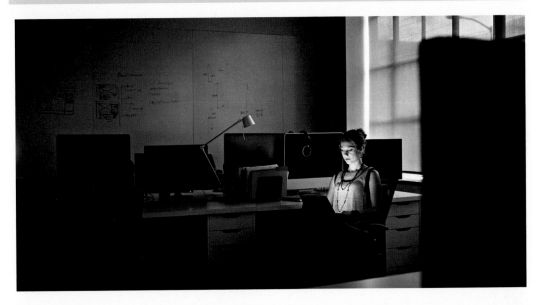

Sleep deprivation is a lack of sleep accumulated over one or several nights. The deprivation may be total, if the sleeper skips a full night of sleep, or partial, if it's limited to the beginning or end of the night.

For experimental purposes, it's possible to deprive subjects selectively of certain specific stages of sleep. Experiments involving the selective deprivation of REM sleep were actually carried out about thirty years ago with depressed patients to see its effects on mood (Chapter 6). This experiment had an antidepressant effect on many patients after several weeks, similar to the effect of antidepressant medications in use at the time. Experiments involving the selective deprivation of slow wave sleep have also been conducted, in order to study the impact of sleep on metabolism (Chapter 5).

After sleep deprivation, the organism tries to catch up and "reimburse its sleep debt." As a result, the nights following sleep deprivation are marked by a rebound in slow wave sleep: there is more of it and sleepers' brain activity shows many slow delta waves (Figure 44). To completely recover from the loss of a full night's sleep, however, it takes more than one night: roughly three nights are required to get over a sleepless night. The first night after a complete night of sleep deprivation is the most restorative and consists largely of slow wave sleep, which decreases gradually over the following nights.

There is also a rebound in REM sleep. After a night of full or partial sleep deprivation, this rebound explains why dreams are more intense during the night of recovery. Since slow wave sleep is more concentrated early in the night and REM sleep is more concentrated at the end of the night, the effect of partial sleep deprivation differs depending on whether it occurs early or late in the night.

Sleep Inertia

When we wake up, it takes us a while to come to. During this transition period, our faculties are weak, our reactions are slower, and our senses are not as sharp. Just as it takes a while to get to sleep, it also takes time to wake up!

This condition, called sleep inertia, depends on the stage of sleep we are in when awakened and on the time of day (Silva and Duffy, 2008). Sleep inertia can be compared to the inertia of a body in motion. The heavier and faster the body in motion is (for example, a train loaded with passengers going full speed), the greater the distance and braking power required to stop it.

Similarly, the deeper the sleep, the greater the confusion during a forced awakening and the more time it takes to become fully awake. Parents of a newborn, doctors on call, firefighters, and members of any emergency team know all about this. We must wait until the inertia has passed before making any important decision that might affect our own safety or someone else's.

Just how big a problem this is appears to vary from one sleeper to another. Some people, especially those who don't "sleep like a log," seem to wake up more easily than others. In comparison, other sleepers take longer to wake up and are sleepier and slower when awakened.

THE EFFECT OF A NIGHT OF SLEEP DEPRIVATION

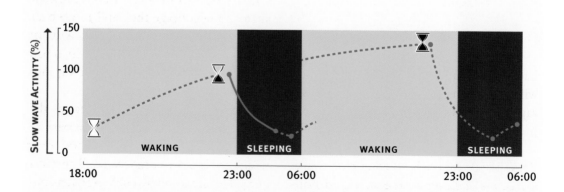

After a night of sleep deprivation, more sand will have built up. The sand will flow more vigorously during the night of recovery, causing more slow wave sleep.

FIGURE 44

Adapted from Borbély et al., 1982.

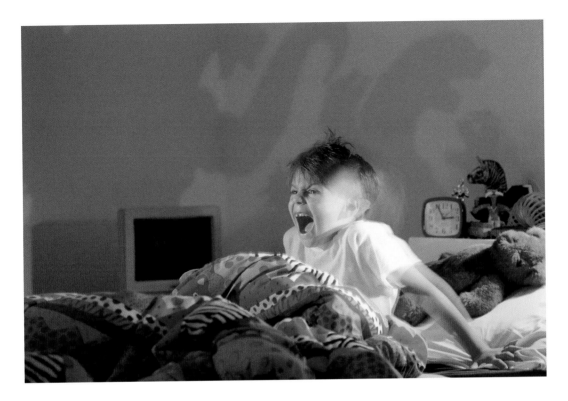

episodes of sleepwalking in patients who are predisposed to them.

NIGHT TERRORS

Night terrors cause a sleeper to wake up in a panic and are usually accompanied by bad dreams and screaming. The sleeper will show signs of anxiety: a faster pulse, rapid breathing, sweating, and dilated pupils. Night terrors, like sleepwalking attacks, occur during stages of non-REM sleep, especially during slow wave sleep, and belong to the so-called non-REM parasomnias. They are therefore more frequent early in the night. Sleepers may seem confused and hard to console at the time. Children are more likely to have night terrors. Once woken up and soothed, children might say in a confused way that they had a bad dream. In fact, the kind of dream and the description sleepers can give of it vary depending on the stage of sleep they awake from. The best attitude for parents to take is to offer reassurance and encourage the child to go back to sleep — in the child's own bed and not the parents' — to avoid getting into bad habits and using night terrors as a way into the parents' bedroom.

Night terrors usually disappear as the child gets older. When they persist or appear for the first time in adulthood, their treatment is more complicated. The possibility that stress and psychological tensions are being expressed in the form of night terrors during sleep must be considered, especially if they are frequent. The possibility that other diagnoses might explain these episodes of nighttime restlessness must also be explored.

HYPNOGRAM SHOWING THE TIMING OF NIGHT TERRORS

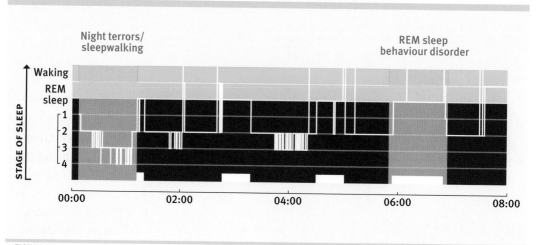

FIGURE 45

Hypnogram, Dr. D.B. Boivin's laboratory.

REM SLEEP BEHAVIOUR DISORDER

REM sleep is a period of heightened brain activity (almost as much as in the waking state), rapid eye movements and loss of muscle tone — total temporary paralysis of the skeletal muscles. A neurological disorder affecting the brain mechanisms responsible for muscle paralysis during REM sleep has been described and is called REM sleep behaviour disorder. The condition involves episodes of nocturnal restlessness and violent behaviours during sleep (Boeve, 2010). Patients awakened after these episodes often report having a restless dream where they were struggling, defending themselves against an enemy, running, or moving around frantically. In reality, they are observed to be restless during sleep, may hit their bed partner, move objects around, hurt themselves, and wake up with bruises on their body and even broken bones.

This disorder is similar to the one described in cats by Professor Michel Jouvet in 1965. At that time, Jouvet's team created an experimental model with the goal of understanding the neurological bases of the temporary muscle paralysis occurring normally during REM sleep. To test the model, the researchers deliberately damaged those parts of the cats' brain stems that cause a loss of muscle tone during REM sleep. The cats injured in this way showed fear, defence, and attack behaviours during their phases of REM sleep, and it was even possible to understand, based on the animals' behaviour, the dreams they were having. We now view this as a good animal model of REM sleep behaviour disorder, although at the time this illness was unknown (Figure 46).

REM sleep behaviour disorder is an intrinsic sleep disorder calling for assessment in a specialized clinic. A polysomnographic study of sleep will reveal the presence of sleep cycles disrupted by periods of abnormal REM sleep. These periods are abnormal because they do not include the loss of muscle tone usually seen during this stage

Dreams

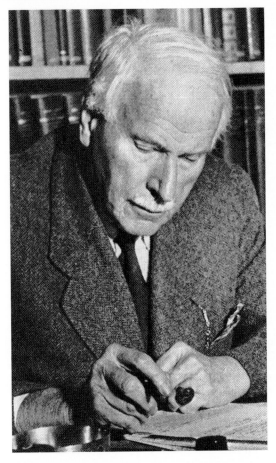

waking and sleeping. During stage 1 sleep, thoughts begin to deviate from reality and the sleeper settles calmly into a dream state. Some people awakened during stage 1 will insist they haven't slept! However, when a full minute has gone by in this stage, the patient is considered to have been asleep. Then comes stage 2, the stage that is the very basis of sleep. In adults, stories of dreams are reported in only about 15 percent of awakenings during this stage, compared with 85 percent for awakenings during the stages of REM sleep.

Recollections of dreams following awakenings from slow wave sleep are harder to obtain, since confusion, and even temporary amnesia, is typical of awakenings from stages 3 and 4 sleep. Dream narratives, if they can be obtained, are much vaguer and less developed than those about dreams that occur during REM sleep. Dream narratives obtained upon awakenings from REM sleep are often complex bizarre stories, with rich visual images and a sequence that is apparently logical to the dreamer, but may be less so to others. When dreams are by nature unpleasant, they are called nightmares. Since there is more REM sleep at the end of the night, nightmares are also more concentrated at that time, compared with night terrors, which occur mainly at the beginning of the night.

Broadly speaking, a dream is any mental imagery occurring during sleep. The type of dream, or at least what the sleeper tells us about it, will differ depending on the stage of sleep when the dream occurs. If we consider the various stages of sleep and their sequence during the night, we first encounter light stage 1 sleep, a transitional phase between

↖ Swiss doctor, psychiatrist, and psychologist Carl G. Jung did major studies on dreams.

of sleep. REM sleep behaviour disorder affects approximately 0.5 percent of the population, especially older men, although women can also have it. It can be associated with other degenerative neurological diseases like Parkinson's disease, or Lewy Body dementia (Postuma et al., 2009). The disorder is treated with medications like clonazepam, which belongs to the class of benzodiazepines, or other medications that act on the nervous system. Therapeutic success using melatonin has recently been reported, but the reasons for its effectiveness as a treatment are not yet understood. When this disorder is caused

by the use of medications (including some used in psychiatry), a clear improvement is seen when they are withdrawn. The safety of the bedroom must also be looked at to minimize the risk of injury for both patient and partner.

NOCTURNAL EPILEPSY

Epilepsy is a disease characterized by sudden convulsive seizures, spasms affecting the arms, legs, and torso. These may affect the entire body, with loss of consciousness and convulsions. They often start in an arm or leg and spread quickly throughout the whole body. This is known as a generalized grand mal seizure. Patients frequently experience urinary incontinence and bite their tongue during these episodes. Sometimes these seizures occur during sleep, and sometimes some patients only have nocturnal seizures (Husain and Sinha, 2011). A history of convulsions during sleep, tongue-biting, and urinary incontinence is an alarm signal that requires medical intervention.

Slow wave sleep is an ideal stage for the spread of epileptic activity to several regions of the brain, whereas seizures tend to be less frequent during periods of REM sleep (the loss of muscle tone means they can't be physically acted out). Some types of epilepsy occurring during waking periods have been described as very complex and associated with bizarre behaviours. This is what happens, for example, in the case of injuries to the temporal regions of the brain. Behaviours of this kind can occur during sleep, without convulsions, but they may also be evidence of epileptic seizures. These are

BRAIN DAMAGE AND REM SLEEP BEHAVIOUR DISORDER

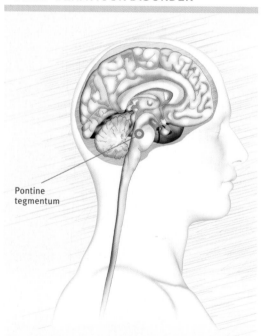

Pontine
tegmentum

According to the Jouvet's model experiment on cats, damage to the pontine tegmentum appears to cause a loss of muscle tone during REM sleep.

FIGURE 46

→ A famous engraving by Spanish painter Francisco de Goya (1746–1828): *The Sleep of Reason Produces Monsters.*

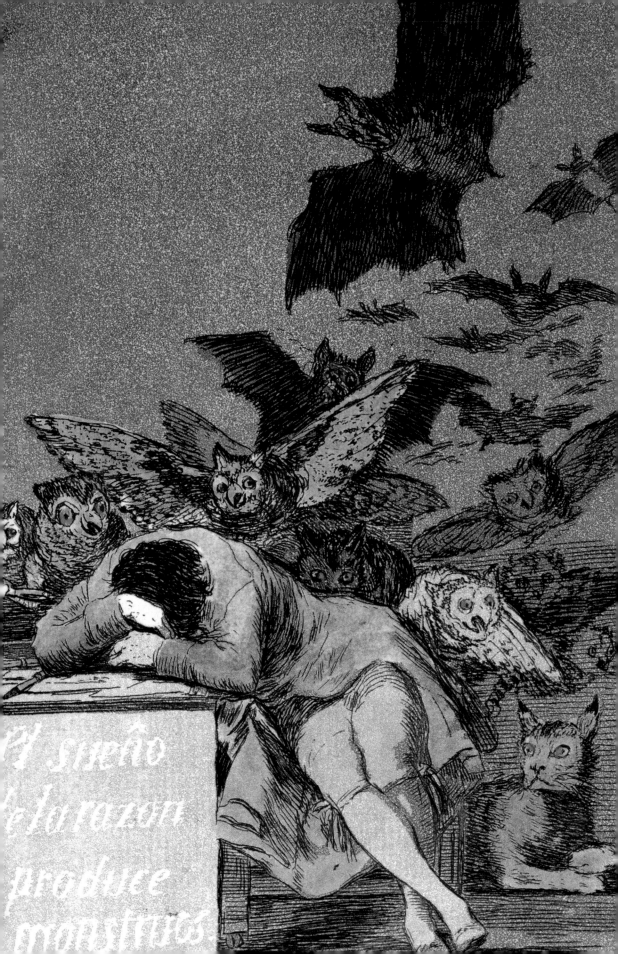

among the most difficult sleep disorders to diagnose, sometimes requiring several polysomnographic studies in a sleep lab. Nocturnal epilepsy is controlled with pharmacological treatment and thus requires antiepileptic medications.

RESTLESS LEGS SYNDROME AND PERIODIC LEG MOVEMENTS DURING SLEEP

Restless legs syndrome (RLS) is a neurological disease in which unpleasant sensations in the arms and legs cause an urgent need to move them around. The sensations are most often felt in the legs, but can also occur in the arms. These unpleasant sensations are described by patients as an impression of heaviness, pins and needles, tingling, burning, or pain. They have a tendency to reach their peak in the evening and early in the night and often make it hard to go to sleep. The unpleasant sensations can be reduced by moving the legs, massage, and walking.

Restless legs syndrome is often associated with periodic leg movements during sleep (PLMS). Patients with this disorder experience repetitive leg movements according to very specific frequency criteria (Figure 47). The repetitive leg movements that occur during sleep disrupt it, reducing its effectiveness and often causing nighttime awakenings. It isn't uncommon for patients to be awakened by their legs and to have to get up and walk so as to alleviate the unpleasant sensations. Sleep-maintenance insomnia often results from this medical disorder. That said, patients are not always aware that they are moving their legs while sleeping; they don't understand why they wake up more tired than when they went to bed and continue to feel tired all day. This is why some patients who have periodic leg movements during sleep report fatigue and daytime sleepiness instead of insomnia.

Restless legs syndrome and periodic leg movements during sleep are two conditions often associated with each other. Until very recently they were considered to be two aspects of the same medical disorder. This is not completely false, since the two disorders have the same biological causes, the same risk factors, and respond to the same treatments. On the other hand, some patients have RLS without PLMS, and others the opposite.

Lastly, some patients have both problems at once. Restless legs syndrome occurs in 5 to 15 percent of the population and is associated with sleep-onset insomnia in 85 percent of cases. It's estimated that roughly 1 to 15 percent of insomniac patients have periodic leg movements during sleep. These are therefore common medical disorders.

These two conditions are related to the inadequate supply of dopamine in the brain stem circuits. In addition, the risk of developing one or the other of these disorders increases with age, as dopamine metabolism

POLYSOMNOGRAPHIC RECORDING OF PERIODIC LEG MOVEMENTS DURING SLEEP (PLMS)

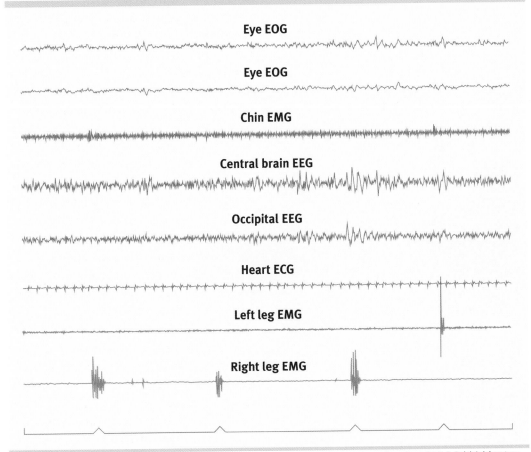

FIGURE 47

Recordings, Dr. D. B. Boivin's laboratory.

deteriorates as we get older. Furthermore, genetic susceptibility factors and the onset of the two syndromes in members of the same family have been observed. Saguenay-Lac-Saint-Jean, in Quebec, is one region where these disorders are very prevalent; this stems from the fact that many marriages in the last century took place within a limited group of people. The result is a susceptibility gene for these diseases. Recent studies have also made it possible to link these conditions to iron deficiency in some regions of the brain, such as the basal ganglia, important for controlling movements. Anemia as well as iron deficiency makes these disorders worse.

The neurological damage at the root of unpleasant sensations in the legs during sleep is located in the brain stem, the part of the nervous system that connects the spinal cord to the brain. The main problem is not therefore in the legs, even though that's where patients feel extremely unpleasant sensations. Back problems and illnesses like kidney failure can make symptoms worse. Patients on

FACTORS AGGRAVATING RLS AND PLMS

- Anemia
- Iron deficiency
- Caffeine
- Alcohol
- Peripheral neuropathies
- Fibromyalgia
- Rheumatoid arthritis
- Sedative antihistamines
- Several antidepressants
- Some antipsychotics

FIGURE 48

renal dialysis can suffer from such a severe case of restless legs syndrome that having to stay still for a long time without moving much becomes a problem for their hemo-dialysis sessions. Some medications and too much caffeine or alcohol can also aggravate these symptoms, making it advisable to limit their consumption (Figure 48).

Restless legs syndrome is diagnosed based on a patient's medical history, while periodic leg movement during sleep is detected using a sleep recording. As the two conditions are often related, doing a polysomnographic study in a sleep lab may be useful. This step makes it possible not only to confirm the diagnosis, but to determine how serious it is.

The discomfort caused by these disorders is treated by medications that reduce the symptoms but do not cure the lifelong disease. This treatment only alleviates the condition, and patients must discuss its advantages and disadvantages with their doctor. Some medications like pramexipole reduce the onset of unpleasant sensations and leg movements during sleep, whereas others like clonezapam reduce the night-time awakenings that go along with it.

In conclusion, the line between waking and sleeping is not always clear, causing some patients to display complex behaviours at night while they are sleeping soundly. Called parasomnias, these phenomena are considered normal in children when they occur during slow wave sleep. They cause problems and often require medical treatment when they continue into adulthood. More serious disorders of a neurological nature, like nocturnal epilepsy or REM sleep behaviour disorder, can also occur. These usually require complex and repeated investigations in a specialized sleep clinic.

What Should You Take
Away From This Chapter?

- Several borderline states of consciousness can be observed during sleep, meaning that sleepers are sleeping deeply but are acting as if they were awake.

- These states, called parasomnias, belong to two main classes: non-REM sleep parasomnias and REM sleep parasomnias.

- Non-REM sleep parasomnias occur mainly at the beginning of the night. This is when sleepwalking and night terrors occur.

- REM-sleep parasomnias occur mainly at the end of the night. This is when REM sleep behaviour disorder occurs.

- Children frequently have non-REM sleep parasomnias, since their sleep consists of a great deal of slow wave sleep.

- Other neurological disorders can occur during the night, like nocturnal epileptic seizures.

- Restless legs syndrome and periodic leg movements during sleep also interfere with sleep efficiency and can cause the patient to get up and walk around at night. These are, however, neurological disorders, not parasomnias.

- Parasomnias in children seldom require pharmacological treatment. However, in adults, serious disorders like REM sleep behaviour disorder, nocturnal epilepsy, and severe periodic leg movements during sleep often require the use of medications.

CONCLUSION

Final Thoughts on Sleep

Sleep is a complex state during which the brain regenerates itself by disconnecting itself from the outside world. This physical and psychological withdrawal allows the neurons to let go of the intense connections they form during the waking period and, in a way, start the new day with a clean slate.

The exact cellular mechanisms causing the brain and body to rest during sleep are only partially understood and are the subject of intense research. The latest discoveries show the important role played by supporting cells in the brain and their communication with neurons in regulating the waking and sleeping states. It's clear that the mechanisms involved in producing sleep and slow wave sleep are intimately related to those involved in brain regeneration. These observations indicate that better sleep and lifestyle hygiene could improve health and, as a result, quality of life in later years.

This knowledge has also resulted in strategies for treating depression based on manipulating the sleep-wake cycle. Studies in this area show that sleeping and not sleeping affect mood and brain regeneration simultaneously. These avenues of research are encouraging as they support the development of advice that takes into account sleep schedules and exposure to light and darkness. These practical interventions can often be used to enhance the beneficial effects of pharmacological treatments.

Sleep also helps us learn and acquire new knowledge. The various stages of sleep that occur in sequence throughout the night form a kind of assembly line for integrating and storing new knowledge acquired the previous day. We can thus retain this knowledge in the long term and perform better as a result if we get proper sleep. As for athletes, it's in their best interest to make good sleep hygiene a part of their training, a piece of advice that's even more pertinent when jet lag is involved! Could a golden sleep mean a golden medal?

Sleeping and waking make up a cycle influenced by the biological clock that controls our body's daily rhythms. The so-called circadian clock controls cycles of roughly twenty-four hours inside our bodies. This central clock decodes environmental signals that tell it what time of day or night it is and in so doing aligns our internal biological day with the terrestrial day. The most powerful of these signals, the alternation of light and darkness, makes sure that even the biological clocks of some blind patients manage to perceive light and adjust to the signal. For this reason, treating all circadian disorders requires rigorous control of exposure to light. Recent research in our laboratory and others has shown that there is more than one circadian clock. We have shown that the desynchronization of these peripheral clocks from each other might play a major role in difficulties in adjusting to night work and lead to increased risk of the onset of certain medical disorders in night workers.

Finally, the past decade has been full of discoveries about the metabolic impacts of sleep and its restriction. Sleep deprivation of even a few hours a night affects sugar and fat metabolism and increases the risk of being overweight: you have to sleep to stay slim! Once the extra pounds have settled in, the risk of developing health problems, including sleep apnea syndrome, increases. Since prevention is better than cure, it would be wise to close down that line of credit at the sleep bank. This could be the start of a trend, for in our modern-day frenetically paced lives, lack of sleep and fatigue, as well as ways of managing them, will remain a favourite subject until we finally get enough sleep, and the subject itself sends us off to dreamland …

About the Author

DR. DIANE B. BOIVIN, MD, PH.D.

Dr. Diane B. Boivin is a Professor of Medicine and Psychiatry at McGill University in Montreal. After completing her medical training in 1986, she chose to continue her academic studies at the Université de Montréal, completing a Ph.D. in neurological sciences, for which she was awarded the Gold Medal of the Governor General of Canada. She then completed a postdoctoral fellowship on human circadian rhythms at Harvard, before returning to Montreal in 1997. She is the founder and director of the Centre for Study and Treatment of Circadian Rhythms at the Douglas Mental Health University Institute.

At the Douglas Institute, Dr. Boivin studies individuals in a time-isolated environment for several days and weeks at a time. Her studies focus on the effect of light on human circadian rhythms, with potential applications for night workers and travellers. Her team and their collaborators were the first to detect rhythms in the circadian clock genes of white blood cells. They have shown that these rhythms can be disrupted at a fundamental level when individuals live on a nocturnal schedule. These results open the door to new and promising avenues of research to help people cope with unconventional work schedules. Dr. Boivin is also interested in the role played by the biological clock in heart function and in the interaction among circadian, menstrual, and seasonal rhythms. Her research is important for understanding the impacts of sleep disruption and circadian rhythms on physical and mental health.

Dr. Boivin is on the editorial committee of a number of major scientific journals: *Sleep, Sleep Medicine, Journal of Biological*

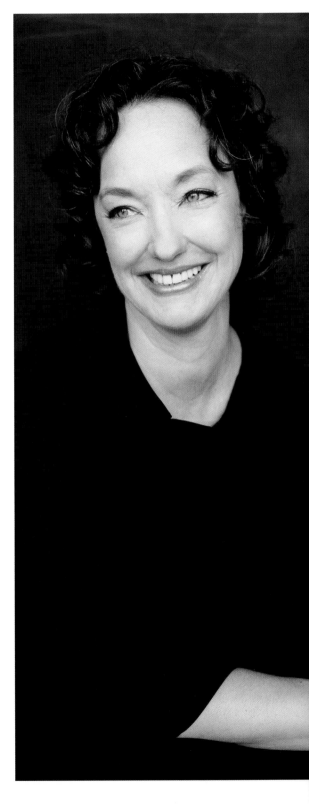

Rhythms, and *Chronobiology International.* In 2007 she was guest editor of a special edition of the journal *Sleep Medicine,* dealing with circadian rhythm disorders, and in 2012 she became associate editor of the journal *Sleep,* one of the most important in the field. Since the beginning of her career, she has authored nearly 300 scientific publications, including research articles, book chapters, books, research reports, and conference summaries. She has also been a member of the science committee for many national and international conferences on sleep. In addition to having a very busy academic career, Dr. Boivin is a lecturer and scientific expert on many subjects related to managing fatigue in the workplace and serves as a medical-legal consultant on litigious cases related to waking and sleeping disorders.

To Learn More ...

CHAPTER 1: Hitting the Sack

Borbély, A.A., and P. Achermann. "Sleep homeostasis and models of sleep regulation." *Journal of Biological Rhythms* 14, no. 6 (1999): 557–68.

Kollar, E.J., R.O. Pasnau, R.T. Rubin, P. Naitoh, G.G. Slater, and A. Kales. "Psychological, psychophysiological, and biochemical correlates of prolonged sleep deprivation." *American Journal of Psychiatry* 126, no. 4 (1969): 488–97.

Luckhaupt, S.E., S. Woo Tak, and G.M. Calvert. "The Prevalence of Short Sleep Duration by Industry and Occupation." In The National Health Interview Survey. *Sleep* 33, no. 2 (2010): 149–59.

Pasnau, R.O., P. Naitoh, S. Stier, and E.J. Kollar. "The Psychological Effects of 205 Hours of Sleep Deprivation." *Archives of General Psychiatry* 18, no. 4 (1968): 496–505.

Saper, C.B., P.M. Fuller, N.P. Pedersen, J. Lu, and T.E. Scammell. "Sleep State Switching." *Neuron* 68, no. 6 (2010): 1023–42, doi:10.1016/j.neuron.2010.11.032.

Tasali, E., R. Leproult, D.A. Ehrmann, et al. "Slow-wave sleep and the risk of type 2 diabetes in humans." *Proceedings of the National Academy of Sciences USA* 105 (2008): 1044–49.

Van Dongen, H.P., M.D. Baynard, G. Maislin, and D. F. Dinges. "Systematic inter-individual differences in neurobehavioral impairment from sleep loss: evidence of trait-like differential vulnerability." *Sleep* 27, no. 3 (2004): 423–33.

Vogel, G.W., F. Vogel, R.S. McAbee, and A.J. Thurmond. "Improvement of depression by REM sleep deprivation: new findings and a theory." *Archives of General Psychiatry* 37, no. 3 (1980): 247–53.

Wagner, U., et al. "Sleep inspires insight." *Nature* 427 (2004): 352–55.

CHAPTER 2: My Planet Earth

Arendt, J. "Managing jet lag: Some of the problems and possible new solutions." *Sleep Medicine Reviews* 13, no. 4 (2009): 249–56.

Barger, L.K., et al. "Impact of extended-duration shifts on medical errors, adverse events, and attentional failures." *PLoS Medicine* 3, no. 12 (2006): 487.

Boivin, D.B., and F.O. James. "Phase dependent effect of room light exposure in a 5-hour advance of the sleep/wake cycle: implications for jet lag." *Journal of Biological Rhythms* 17, no. 3 (2002): 266–76.

Boivin, D.B., G.M. Tremblay, and P. Boudreau. *Les horaires rotatifs chez les policiers : étude des approches préventives complémentaires de réduction de la fatigue.* Montreal: Institut de recherche Robert-Sauvé en santé et en sécurité du travail, 2010.

Brown, S.A., et al. "Molecular insights into human daily behavior." *Proceedings of the National Academy of Sciences USA* 105 (2008): 1602–07.

Cermakian, N., and D.B. Boivin. "A molecular perspective of human circadian rhythm disorders." *Brain Research Reviews* 42, no. 3 (2003): 204–20.

Cuesta, M. "Modulation sérotonergique différentielle de l'horloge circadienne principale entre rongeurs diurnes et nocturnes." Ph.D. Diss., Université de Strasbourg, 2009.

Czeisler, C., T.L. Shanahan, E.B. Klerman, H. Martens, D.J. Brotman, J.S. Emens, T. Klein, and J.F. Rizzo III. "Suppression of melatonin secretion in some blind patients by exposure to bright light." *New England Journal of Medicine* 332, no. 1 (1995): 6–11.

Gronfier, C., K.P. Wright, R.E. Kronauer, and C.A. Czeisler. "Entrainment of the human circadian pacemaker to longer-than-24-h days." *Proceedings of the National Academy of Sciences USA* 104, no. 21 (2007): 9081–86.

Hurst, M. "Who gets any sleep these days? Sleep patterns of Canadians." Ottawa: Statistics Canada 11-008, 2008.

Khalsa, S.B., M.E. Jewett, C. Cajochen, and C.A. Czeisler. "A phase response curve to single bright light pulses in human subjects." *The Journal of Physiology* 549 (2003): 945–52.

Wittmann, M., J. Dinich, M. Merrow, and T. Roenneberg. "Social jet lag: misalignment of biological and social time." *Chronobiology International* 23, nos. 1 and 2 (2006): 497–509.

CHAPTER 3: Searching for the Fountain of Youth

Cain, S., C.F. Dennison, J.M. Zeitzer, A.M. Guzik, S.B.S. Khalsa, N. Santhi, M.W. Schoen, C.A. Czeisler, and J.F. Duffy. "Sex Differences in Phase Angle of Entrainment and Melatonin Amplitude in Humans." *Journal of Biological Rhythms* 25, no. 4 (2010): 288–96.

Carrier. J., I. Viens, G. Poirier, R. Robillard, M. Lafortune, G. Vandewalle, N. Martin, M. Barakat, G. Paquet, and D. Filipini. "Sleep slow wave changes during the middle years of life." *European Journal of Neuroscience* 33, no. 4 (2011): 758–66.

Cermakian, N., E. Waddington-Lamont, P. Boudreau and D.B. Boivin. "Circadian Clock Gene Expression in Brain Regions of Alzheimer's Disease Patients and Control Subjects." *Journal of Biological Rhythms* 26, no. 2 (2011): 160–70.

Duffy, J.F., S.W. Cain, A.-M. Chang, A.J.K. Phillips, M.Y. Münch, C. Gronfier, J.K. Wyatt, D.-J. Dijk, K.P. Wright, Jr., and C.A. Czeisler. "Sex difference in the near-24-hour intrinsic period of the human circadian timing system." *Proceedings of the National Academy of Sciences USA* 108 (2011): 15,602–08.

Hagenauer, M.H., J.I. Perryman, T.M. Lee, and M.A. Carskadon. "Adolescent Changes in the Homeostatic and Circadian Regulation of Sleep." *Developmental Neuroscience* 31, no. 4 (2009): 276–84.

Kurth, S., O.G. Jenni, B.A. Riedner, G. Tononi, M.A. Carskadon, and R. Huber. "Characteristics of sleep slow waves in children and adolescents." *Sleep* 33, no. 4 (2010): 475–80.

Owens, J.A., C. Jones, and R. Nash. "Caregivers' Knowledge, Behavior, and Attitudes Regarding Healthy Sleep in Young Children." *Journal of Clinical Sleep Medicine* 7, no. 4 (2011): 345–50.

Schechter, A., P. L'Espérance, Ng Ying Kin, NMK, and D.B. Boivin. "Nocturnal Polysomnographic Sleep across the Menstrual Cycle in Premenstrual Dysphoric Disorder." *Sleep Medicine* (forthcoming).

Sowers, M.F., H. Zheng, H.M. Kravitz, K. Matthews, J.T. Bromberger, E.B. Gold, J. Owens, F. Consens, and M. Hall. "Sex Steroid Hormone Profiles are Related to Sleep Measures from Polysomnography and the Pittsburgh Sleep Quality Index." *Sleep* 31, no. 10 (2008): 1339–49.

CHAPTER 4: When You Miss the Boat

Budhiraja, R., R. Roth, D.W. Hudgel, P. Budhiraja, and C.L. Drake. "Prevalence and

Polysomnographic Correlates of Insomnia Comorbid with Medical Disorders." *Sleep* 34, no. 7 (2011): 859–67.

Buysse, D.J., J. Angst, A. Gamma, V. Ajdacic, D. Eich, and W. Rössler. "Prevalence, Course, and Comorbidity of Insomnia and Depression in Young Adults." *Sleep* 31, no. 4 (2008): 473–80.

Daley, M., C.M. Morin, M. LeBlanc, J.-P. Grégoire, and J. Savard. "The Economic Burden of Insomnia: Direct and Indirect Costs for Individuals with Insomnia Syndrome, Insomnia Symptoms, and Good Sleepers." *Sleep* 32, no. 1 (2009): 55–64.

McKinstry, B., P. Wilson, and C. Espie. "Non-pharmacological management of chronic insomnia in primary care." *British Journal of General Practice* 58, no. 547 (2008): 79–80.

Palagi, E., A. Leone, G. Mancini, and P. F. Ferrari. "Contagious yawning in gelada baboons as a possible expression of empathy." *Proceedings of the National Academy of Sciences USA* 106, no. 46 (2009): 19,262–67.

Strogatz, S.H., R.E. Kronauer, and C.A. Czeisler. "Circadian pacemaker interferes with sleep onset at specific times each day: role in insomnia." *American Journal of Physiology — Regulatory, Integrative and Comparative Physiology*, 253 (1987): 72–178.

Taylor, D.J., W. Schmidt-Nowara, C.A. Jessop, and J. Ahearn. "Sleep Restriction Therapy and Hypnotic Withdrawal versus Sleep Hygiene Education in Hypnotic Using Patients with Insomnia." *Journal of Clinical Sleep Medicine* 6, no. 2 (2010): 169–75.

Chapter 5: They Who Sleep Forget Their Hunger!

Benedict, C., S.J. Brooks, O.G. O'Daly, M.S. Almen, A. Morell, K. Åberg, M. Gingnell, B. Schultes, M. Hallschmid, J.-E. Broman, E.M. Larsson, and H.B. Schioth. "Acute Sleep Deprivation Enhances the Brain's Response to Hedonic Food Stimuli: An fMRI Study." *Journal of Clinical Endocrinology and Metabolism*, doi:10.1210/jc.2011-2759 (2012).

Boudreau, P., Hsien Yeh Wei, G. Dumont, and D.B. Boivin. "A circadian rhythm in heart rate variability contributes to the increased cardiac sympathovagal response to awakening in the morning." *Chronobiology International* 29, no. 6 (2012): 757–68.

Van Cauter, E., and K.L. Knutson. "Sleep and the epidemic of obesity in children and adults." *European Journal of Endocrinology* 159 (2008): 59–66.

Taveras, E.M., S.L. Rifas-Shiman, E. Oken, E.P. Gunderson, and M.W. Gillman. "Short sleep duration in infancy and risk of childhood overweight." *Archives of Pediatric and Adolescent Medicine* 162, no. 4 (2008): 305–11.

Olcese, U., S.K. Esser, and G. Tononi. "Sleep and Synaptic Renormalization: A Computational Study." *Journal of Neurophysiology* 104, no. 6 (2010): 3,476–93.

Magee, C.A., X.-F. Huang, D.C. Iverson, and P. Caputi. "Examining the Pathways Linking Chronic Sleep Restriction to Obesity." *Journal of Obesity*, article ID 821710, 8 pages, doi:10.1155/2010/821710 (2010).

Dang-Vu, T.T., M. Schabus, M. Desseilles, V. Sterpenich, M. Bonjean, and P. Maquet. "Functional Neuroimaging Insights into the Physiology of Human Sleep." *Sleep* 33, no. 12 (2010): 1,589–1,603.

Chapter 6: Waiting for Prince Charming

Aan het Rot, M., N. Coupland, D.B. Boivin, C. Benkelfat, and S.N. Young. "Recognizing emotions in faces: effects of acute tryptophan depletion and bright light." *Journal of Psychopharmacology* 24, no. 10 (2010): 1,447–54.

Boivin, D.B., C.A. Czeisler, D.J. Dijk, J.F. Duffy, S. Folkard, D. Minors, P. Totterdell, and J. Waterhouse. "Complex interaction of the sleep-wake cycle and circadian phase modulates mood in healthy subjects." *Archives of General Psychiatry* 54, no. 2 (1997): 145–52.

Clark, C.P., G.C. Brown, L. Frank, L. Thomas, A.N. Sutherland, and J.C. Gillin. "Improved anatomic delineation of the antidepressant response to partial sleep deprivation in medial frontal cortex using perfusion-weighted functional MRI." *Psychiatry Research: Neuroimaging*, 146 (2006): 213–22.

Lam, Raymond W., and A.J. Levitt, ed. *Canadian Consensus Guidelines for the Treatment of Seasonal Affective Disorder*. Vancouver: Clinical and Academic Publishing, 1999.

Lewy, A.J., B.J. Lefler, J.S. Emens, and V.K. Bauer. "The Circadian Basis of Winter Depression." *Proceedings of the National Academy of Sciences* 103, no. 19 (2006): 7,414–19.

Magnusson, A., and J. Axelsson. "The Prevalence of Seasonal Affective Disorder Is Low Among Descendants of Icelandic Emigrants in Canada." *Archives of General Psychiatry*: 50 (1993): 947–51.

Rosenthal, N.E., et al. "Seasonal affective disorder. A Description of the Syndrome and Preliminary Findings With Light Therapy." *Archives of General Psychiatry* 41 (1984): 72–80.

Wehr, T.A., and A. Wirz-Justice. "Internal coincidence model for sleep deprivation and depression." In *Sleep,* ed. W.P. Koella (1981), 26–33. Basel: Karger, 1980.

Chapter 7: The Sleeping Beauty

Schwartz, S., A. Ponz, R. Poryazova, E. Werth, P. Boesiger, R. Khatami, and C.L. Bassetti. "Abnormal activity in hypothalamus and amygdala during humour processing in human narcolepsy with cataplexy." *Brain* 131 (2008): 514–22.

Johns, M.W. "A new method for measuring daytime sleepiness: the Epworth Sleepiness Scale." *Sleep* 14, no. 6 (1991): 540–45.

Billiard, M., I. Jaussent, Y. Dauvilliers, and A. Besset. "Recurrent hypersomnia: a review of 339 cases." *Sleep Medicine Review* 15, no. 4 (2011): 247–57.

Dantz, B., D.M. Edgar, and W.C. Dement. "Circadian Rhythms in Narcolepsy: studies on a 90 minute day." *Electroencephalography and Clinical Neurophysiology* 90, no. 1 (1994): 24–35.

Dauvilliers, Y., M. Billiard, and J. Montplaisir. "Clinical Aspects and Pathopsychology of Narcolepsy." *Clinical Neurophysiology* 114 (2003): 2,000–17.

Gélineau, J. "De la narcolepsie." *Gazette des hôpitaux (Paris)*: 53 (1880): 626–28.

Nishino, S., M. Okuro, N. Kotorii, E. Anegawa, Y. Ishimaru, M. Matsumura, and T. Kanbayashi. "Hypocretin/orexin and narcolepsy: new basic and clinical insights." *Acta Physiologica* (Oxford) 198, no. 3 (2010): 209–22.

Vernet, C., and I. Arnulf. "Idiopathic Hypersomnia with and without Long Sleep Time: A Controlled Series of 75 Patients." *Sleep* 32, no. 6 (2009): 753–59.

Chapter 8: An Unexpected Climb up Mount Everest

Fleetham, J., N. Ayas, D. Bradley, K. Ferguson, M. Fitzpatrick, C. George, P. Hanly, F. Hill, J. Kimoff, M. Kryger, D. Morrison, F. Series, and W. Tsai. "Directives de la Société canadienne de thoracologie: Diagnostic et traitement des troubles respiratoires du sommeil de l'adulte." *Canadian Respiratory Journal* 14, no (2007). 1: 31–36.

Jean-Louis, G., F. Zizi, L.T. Clark, C.D. Brown, and S.I. McFarlane. 2008. "Obstructive Sleep Apnea and Cardiovascular Disease: Role of the Metabolic Syndrome and Its Components." *Journal of Clinical Sleep Medicine* 4, no. 3: 261–72.

Schwartz, A.R., S.P. Patil, A.M. Laffan, V. Polotsky, H. Schneider, and P. Smith. "Obesity and Obstructive Sleep Apnea: Pathogenic Mechanisms and Therapeutic Approaches." *Proceedings of the American Thoracic Society* 5, no. 2 (2008): 185–92.

Micheli, K., I. Komninos, E. Bagkeris, T. Roumeliotaki, A. Koutis, M. Kogevinas, and L. Chatzi. "Sleep patterns in late pregnancy and risk of preterm birth and fetal growth restriction." *Epidemiology* 22, no. 5 (2011): 738–44.

Lal, C., C. Strange, and D. Bachman. "Neurocognitive impairment in obstructive sleep apnea." *Chest* 141, no. 6 (2012): 1,601–10.

Bulcun, E., M. Ekici, and A. Ekici. "Disorders of glucose metabolism and insulin resistance in patients with obstructive sleep apnoea syndrome." *International Journal of Clinical Practice* 66, no. 1 (2012): 91–97.

Heinzer, R.C., C. Pellaton, V. Rey, A.O. Rossetti, G. Lecciso, J. Haba-Rubio, M. Tafti, and G. Lavigne. "Positional therapy for obstructive sleep apnea: an objective measurement of patients' usage and efficacy at home." *Sleep Medicine* 13, no. 4 (2012): 425–28.

CHAPTER 9: Bedtime Stories

Jouvet, M., and F. Delorme. "Locus coeruleus et sommeil paradoxal." *Comptes rendus des séances de la Société de Biologie et de ses filiales* 159 (1965): 895–99.

Boeve, B.F. "REM Sleep Behavior Disorder: Updated Review of the Core Features, The RBD-Neurodegenerative Disease Association, Evolving Concepts, Controversies, and Future Directions." *Annals of the New York Academy of Sciences* 1,184 (2010): 15–54.

Postuma, R.B., J.F. Gagnon, M. Vendette, M.L. Fantini, J. Massicotte-Marquez, and J. Montplaisir. "Quantifying the risk of neurodegenerative disease in idiopathic REM sleep behavior disorder." *Neurology* 72, no. 15 (2009): 1,296–300.

Mahowald, M.W., M.A. Cramer Bornemann, and C.H. Schenck. "State dissociation, human behavior, and consciousness." *Current Topics in Medicinal Chemistry* 11, no. 19 (2011): 2,392–402.

Umanath, S., D. Sarezky, and S. Finger. "Sleepwalking through history: medicine, arts, and courts of law." *Journal of Historical Neuroscience* 20, no. 4 (2011): 253–76.

Cao, M., and C. Guilleminault. "Families with sleepwalking." *Sleep Medicine* 11, no. 7 (2010): 726–34.

Silva, E.J., and J.F. Duffy. "Sleep inertia varies with circadian phase and sleep stage in older adults." *Behavioral Neuroscience* 122, no. 4 (2008): 928–35.

Husain, A.M., and S.R. Sinha. "Nocturnal epilepsy in adults." *Journal of Clinical Neurophysiology* 28, no. 2 (2011): 141–45.

IMAGE CREDITS

JASMIN GUÉRARD-ALIE: 16, 40, 58, 72, 88, 100, 116, 132, 148

AMÉLIE ROBERGE: 33, 35, 36, 42, 48, 49, 69, 96, 107, 125, 126, 135, 136, 144, 158

GETTY IMAGES: Denise Balyoz Photography/Flickr/Getty Images couverture; Marion Peck/Illustration Works/Getty Images 15; Time Life Pictures/Getty Images 18; Ghislain & Marie David de Lossy/The Agency Collection/Getty Images 19; Thomas Kokta/Woorkbook Stock/Getty Images 22; Laurence Monneret/StockImage/Getty Images 24; UpperCut Images/Getty Images 26; Bruno Brunelli/Fototrove/Getty Images 28; Tyler Stableford/Iconica/Getty Images 30; Kevin Morris/Stone/Getty Images 31; Mark Tyacke VisionAiry Photography/Flickr/Getty Images 34; HANK MORGAN/Photo Researchers/Getty Images 37; Les Stocker/Oxford Scientific/Getty Images 43 (left); Andrew JK Tan/Flickr/Getty Images 43 (right); Christian Beirle González/Flickr/Getty Images 44; Lucy Lambriex/Flickr/Getty Images 47; Ian Gethings/Flickr/Getty Images 51; Paul Bradbury/OJO Images/Getty Images 53; Eric CHRETIEN/Gamma-Rapho/Getty Images 54; Fuse/Getty Images 55; Ron Levine/The Image Bank/Getty Images 60; Fuse/Getty Images 61; Ranald Mackechnie/Stockbyte/Getty Images 63 (left); Reza Estakhrian/Stone/Getty Images 63 (right); Margo Silver/Taxi/Getty Images 64; Anthony Nagelmann/UpperCut Images 65; Ben Ivory/Flickr Select/Getty Images 67; Rubberball Productions/Getty Images 68; Photodisc/Getty Images 76; Dave O Tuttle/Flickr/Getty Images 78; Anne Rippy/The Image Bank/Getty Images 79; Alexandra Grablewski/Lifesize/Getty Images 80; R. Brandon Harris/Flickr/Getty Images 82; PM Images/The Image Bank/Getty Images 83; Betsie Van der Meer/Stone/Getty Images 84; Scimat Scimat/Photo Researchers/Getty Images 85; Betsie Van der Meer/Stone/Getty Images 86; Digital Vision/Getty Images 90; Tetra Images/Getty Images 94; susan.k./Flickr/Getty Images 95; Coco McCoy-Rainbow/Science Faction/Getty Images 104; Infocus International/The Image Bank/Getty Images 106; Jacqueline Veissid/Photodisc/Getty Images 109; Dave Greenwood/Taxi/Getty Images 110; (c) Jaime Monfort/Flickr/Getty Images 119; Eric Audras/ONOKY/Getty Images 120; Henry Fuseli/The Bridgeman Art Library 123; Tanya Constantine/Blend Images/Getty Images 124; Photodisc/Getty Images 127; Paul Bradbury/OJO Images/Getty Images 128; Ian Shive/Aurora/Getty Images 134; David Madison/Photographer's Choice 137; David Trood/Stone+/Getty Images 138; Stockbyte/Getty Images 139; Altrendo Images/Altrendo/Getty Images 140; Steven Puetzer/Workbook Stock/Getty Images 143; Ron Koeberer/Aurora/Getty Images 151; Jekaterina Nikitina/Flickr/Getty Images 152; Thomas Barwick/Iconica/Getty Images 153; Zigy Kaluzny/Stone/Getty Images 155; SCIENCE SOURCE/Photo Researchers/Getty Images 157; Francisco Jose de Goya y Lucientes/The Bridgeman Art Library/Getty Images 159; IAN HOOTON/SPL/Science Photo Library/Getty Images 160

SHUTTERSTOCK: 97

SARAH SCOTT: 176

CONTACT INFORMATION

DR DIANE B. BOIVIN
Centre d'étude et de traitement des rythmes circadiens
Institut universitaire en santé mentale Douglas
6875, boul. Lasalle
Montréal (Québec) H4H 1R3
Canada

Telephone: 514 761-6131
Fax: 514 888-4099
www.douglasresearch.qc.ca/circadian

Also in the Your Health Series

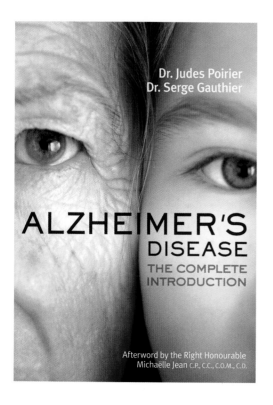

ALZHEIMER'S DISEASE
The Complete Introduction
By Dr. Judes Poirier and
Dr. Serge Gauthier

Alzheimer's disease is a reality in millions of lives and a serious concern for seniors and their loved ones. In developed countries where people are living longer than ever before, the incidence of Alzheimer's is reaching epidemic proportions, according to the World Health Organization. For families, sufferers, and caregivers, the need for reliable, clear, and concrete information has never been greater.

Alzheimer's Disease: The Complete Introduction is a comprehensive guide to the disease and its effects: getting a diagnosis, the ways it can progress and be managed, strategies for supporting sufferers and accessing care, legal concerns, and more. This guide addresses every aspect of the disease from the first doctor's visit to the long-term measures that can drastically improve the lives of sufferers and those close to them.

Coming in January 2015

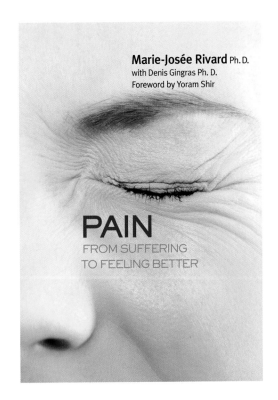

PAIN
From Suffering to Feeling Better
By Marie-Josée Rivard, Ph.D.
with Denis Gingras, Ph.D.

Pain strikes all of us, but it becomes a recurring or constant condition for one in five people. For millions, young and old, it is a difficult, day-to-day reality, and many sufferers have been left feeling more frustrated and helpless than ever, despite medical advances.

Pain is a guide to understanding and treating all kinds of pain, and helping sufferers maintain hope for a normal life. In accessible chapters, this book explains how pain occurs at a fundamental level, both psychologically and physically, and what makes ordinary pain debilitating.

Available at your favourite bookseller

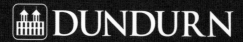

DUNDURN

Visit us at
Dundurn.com
@dundurnpress
Facebook.com/dundurnpress
Pinterest.com/dundurnpress